COPING WITH LYME DISEASE

COPING WITH LYME DISEASE

COPING WITH
LYME
DISEASE

A Practical Guide to Dealing with Diagnosis and Treatment

THIRD EDITION

DENISE LANG

with Kenneth B. Liegner, M.D.
Foreword by Mary McDonnell

AN OWL BOOK
HENRY HOLT AND COMPANY   NEW YORK

Owl Books
Henry Holt and Company, LLC
Publishers since 1866
175 Fifth Avenue
New York, New York 10010
www.henryholt.com

An Owl Book® and ⬡® are registered trademarks of
Henry Holt and Company, LLC.

Library of Congress Cataloging-in-Publication Data
Lang, Denise V.
    Coping with lyme disease : a practical guide to dealing with
diagnosis and treatment / Denise Lang, with Kenneth B. Liegner.—3rd ed.
        p.   cm.
    Includes bibliographical references and index.
    ISBN-13: 978-0-8050-7563-2
    ISBN-10: 0-8050-7563-1
    1. Lyme disease—Popular works.   I. Liegner, Kenneth B.   II. Title.
RC155.5.L38 2004
616.9'246—dc22   2003067772

Henry Holt books are available for special promotions and
premiums. For details contact: Director, Special Markets.

First Edition 1993
Second Edition 1997
Third Edition 2004

Printed in the United States of America

5   7   9   10   8   6   4

For Christopher
Who fought with strength and persistence . . . and won!

Contents

III.
GETTING TREATMENT AND SUPPORT

Foreword

Several years ago, I started hearing from relatives that my cousin Pat Loughran was losing her husband Jim to the ravages of Lyme disease. The notion that Jim might die from this thing called Lyme disease was simultaneously deeply disturbing and vaguely unreal to me.

I had been through the excruciating experience of watching friends and family members struggle with, and in some cases lose the battle to disease (cancer, AIDS, Alzheimer's, heart disease, etc.). My response to these situations was always distinct and vivid. My response to Jim's situation had a numbness to it, a kind of distance that I did not understand.

When Jim did eventually die from Lyme, I felt alarmed and very, very angry. Why and how was it possible that this beautiful man could be gone and his family robbed of his life from something so innocuous as a tick bite?

I now recognize my response as common to the early stages of understanding Lyme. My reaction was rooted in ignorance. We as a society are deeply afraid of confronting a disease that can come upon us quietly and without warning, in our most natural and peaceful environments.

Every man, woman, and child who has fallen victim to Lyme, and every member of their devoted families has had to confront this dark and mysterious illness with herculean amounts of tenacity and courage. And so it was, and still is, with my cousin Pat, a remarkable woman possessing the faith and energy of ten women.

Pat invited me to help her and hundreds of others in their noble endeavor to create Lyme disease awareness. And so began the last few years of my being privileged to meet and witness the extraordinary people who are using every spare moment of their lives in the effort to identify, treat, and someday, against all odds, discover the cure for this confounding disease. What I have found in the people who are fighting Lyme is a deep conviction in the preservation of life, a passionate commitment to saving the lives of thousands of children, and a relentless willingness to chip away at the layers of bureaucracy and politics that impede the possibility of cure.

In the following pages, Denise Lang compassionately and practically offers invaluable insight into the world of Lyme. She invites us, with a certainty that comes only through the personal journey of a loving parent, into a world that in her deft hands feels not so vague, not so threatening, and ultimately full of hope.

I am deeply honored to be a part of this truly significant book. I invite you to read it cover to cover, and I implore you to give the book to others. Eventually, if not already, you will know someone afflicted with Lyme. Give that person this book. It is possible that you will help save his or her life.

In *Coping with Lyme Disease,* Denise Lang bridges the world of torment that confuses and exhausts the Lyme sufferer, to a world of information, understanding, and, at long last, relief. What a treasure this book is. Bravo, and thank you, Denise.

MARY MCDONNELL, ACTRESS
NATIONAL SPOKESPERSON,
LYME DISEASE ASSOCIATION, INC. (LDA)

COPING WITH LYME DISEASE

Introduction

Soft ocean breezes wafted inland as I sat in the standing-room-only auditorium of Westerly Hospital, in Westerly, Rhode Island, in August of 2002, awaiting the start of an unusual informational seminar on Lyme disease.

Some of the most knowledgeable physicians and activists were scheduled to speak, but we were also to hear from members of the Governor's Commission on Lyme Disease—a committee deemed necessary when Rhode Island moved ahead of New Jersey to win the dubious distinction of having the second-highest infection rate in the country. An underlying current of tension permeated what would otherwise have been a lighthearted summer day.

A lovely but worried looking brunette sat down next to me and extended her hand.

"You're Denise Lang. You wrote the book *Coping with Lyme Disease*, didn't you? Well, you should talk to me. I just had to sell all my living room and dining room furniture to pay for antibiotics for my two kids."

Tears welled in her eyes.

"My husband and I have worked hard all our lives, paid our insurance premiums, tried to be good citizens. But now, when we need help . . . well, I'm not sure how much more furniture I can sell. And without the antibiotics, my kids will get really sick. My husband has it, too, but we can't afford to treat him. Some days, I just get really scared."

In those few short moments, a dozen years flashed before my eyes.

When I wrote the first edition of *Coping with Lyme Disease,* it was in the wake of my then-teenage son's descent into the hell that Lyme can bring upon a family. Ten months of misdiagnosis and being shuffled from specialist to specialist. Ten months of watching a bright, optimistic, and able honors student detcriorate into a shaking, pain-wracked, and depressed boy who whispered as we sat at a traffic light following another unfruitful doctor's visit, "If I have to spend the rest of my life like this, I don't know that it's worth living."

Ten months of financial drain, family tension, sleepless nights, and desperation that eventually contributed to the erosion of my marriage. Ten months of fighting for credibility with doctors, fighting for calm in the face of helplessness, and fighting for the sanity to go on.

And then—finally—a diagnosis and treatment. Successful, long-term treatment, I should add.

All of that flashed through my head in a nanosecond in the face of this upset woman, yet the first conscious thought that popped to mind was, "I thought by now, things would be different."

The fact of the matter is things *are* different from the time of publication of the first edition of this book in 1993 and even the 1997 update. Some of those differences are good, and some are not so good.

The good news is that many more doctors, nurses, scientists, and legislators are aware of Lyme disease and how it can infect the lives of more than just the patient. The Centers for Disease Control (CDC) finally acknowledges the existence of chronic Lyme disease and cautions, in writing, that generally only one out of ten cases is reported—particularly startling when you consider that cases of *reported* Lyme hit 23,764 in 2002. And the Surgeon General stated as a goal in *Healthy People 2010* to reduce Lyme disease cases by 44 percent in endemic areas.

The bad news is that people in many parts of the country still have to fight for a diagnosis, and too many doctors who are successfully treating Lyme disease have been harassed by ignorant medical boards acting under pressure from insurance companies that don't want to pay for costly medication.

The good news is that the studies, peer-reviewed articles, and research that will enable doctors and scientists to understand, diagnose, and treat Lyme have been, and continue to be, produced. The bad news is that Lyme has now been confounded by a whole host of other tick-borne infections, further complicating an already difficult diagnosis.

The good news is that there is much more information available—on the Internet, through support groups, and from organizations such as the Lyme Disease Association and the International Lyme and Associated Diseases Society (a professional medical and research organization)—than ever before. The bad news is that they still have to fight popular, academic, and governmental ignorance to reach the people who need their help.

And the good news is that they are continuing to fight—for you and for me.

Some of you are veterans of the war on Lyme and will notice that some passages in this book have remained the same, while others have changed dramatically. Some of you are reading this book for the first time because someone you know and love has Lyme, has been touched by Lyme, or is struggling for a diagnosis of an as-yet unnamed illness. My hope is that you will consider the information in this book—garnered from some of the top experts in the country—as another educational tool as you become a savvy medical consumer.

And that's the most hopeful change over the past dozen years: we now know that we have to think like *medical consumers*— not patients, victims, or docile sponges—educating ourselves and demanding the same quality of care for ourselves that we would expect for our prized sports car.

Whatever your situation, know that you *can* beat Lyme disease with varying success—another wonderful change—and that you are *not* alone!

I.

RECOGNIZING THE

VARIED ASPECTS

OF LYME DISEASE

1.

Lyme Disease: The Cost in Human Terms

Lyme disease has emerged as a threat to public health worldwide. It is a particularly vexing problem in the United States, where it is growing in range and intensity. In fact, in some regions, it is now such a threat that it interferes with all sorts of outdoor activities and has even led to depreciation of real estate values.

—Dr. Robert Edelman, professor of medicine and associate director for Clinical Research at the Center for Vaccine Development, University of Maryland School of Medicine

They can tell you to the day—sometimes to the hour—the last time they felt well. These patients who have suffered debilitating symptoms and numerous losses: of jobs, school years, families, relationships, self-esteem, and financial stability. They blame not only the disease but the plethora of doctors who didn't listen, wouldn't believe, or passed them along to other physicians when the diagnosis for this epidemic illness was too challenging. And they are very angry.

The doctors, too, are angry and can't tell you the last time they practiced medicine with the purity and curiosity of spirit inspired by the Hippocratic oath. Some still do, in the face of ridicule from more cynical or sheltered colleagues. And some, who have themselves been victims of this disease—bombarded with tests, interrogations, and skepticism from peers—now view their colleagues in a different light and speak in terms of having to "fight this war" at any cost.

This is the face of Lyme disease.

Once considered only a minor irritation in the northeastern United States, Lyme disease has spread to forty-nine states and eighty countries across six continents, and its pathology embodies some of the medical profession's worst nightmares regarding diagnosis and treatment. The most commonly reported tickborne systemic illness, Lyme disease has been called the fastest-growing epidemic of the twentieth century, now surpassing AIDS. While, unlike AIDS, Lyme disease is rarely listed as a direct cause of death, misdiagnosis and delay in treatment can lead to permanent disability since the infectious spirochete that causes the disease has an affinity for lodging in, and destroying, major systems of the human body—including the central nervous system, where it evades most antibiotics. It has now also been documented as able to hide in the cells and change its presentation, in much the same way as a clever and lethal thief, because its complex life cycle includes a cystic form that resists antibiotics. When the "coast is clear," the spirochetal form then reemerges to wreak havoc on the poor victim's bodily systems.

Lyme disease is therefore frequently referred to as a disease of morbidity (or sickness) rather than mortality, but it is more than that. If promptly diagnosed and treated aggressively with antibiotics, Lyme disease, theoretically, can be cured, although there is no existing test that will confirm a cured state. However, if, because of its widely confusing symptoms, diagnosis and treatment are delayed, it can become a chronic disease of debilitation—physical, mental, and social debilitation. At the extreme, Lyme is blamed for a growing number of suicides among those infected.

So what exactly is the problem? In this age of fast food and modern medical miracles, why can't physicians consider the symptoms, order supportive tests, and begin treatment promptly? The answer promises to inspire a medical Armageddon so all-encompassing that the legal system, the insurance industry, public health agencies, educational systems, and government entities are all being forced to reevaluate traditionally accepted paradigms.

THE SPREAD OF LYME DISEASE

The story of Lyme disease as we know it in the United States began in 1975, when two mothers, alarmed by a rash of cases of joint inflammation in their communities of Lyme and East Haddam, Connecticut, contacted public health authorities. Research scientists at Yale University, headed by Dr. Allen Steere and supported by the National Institute of Arthritis and Musculoskeletal and Skin Diseases, identified what was first known as "Lyme arthritis" in thirty-nine children and twelve adults. Since then, the disease has proven to be more ubiquitous than at first thought.

In 1978 Dr. Steere's team discovered that the disease was being transmitted by the bite of the *Ixodes dammini* tick. In 1981 Dr. Willy Burgdorfer and his colleagues at the Rocky Mountain Laboratories of the National Institute of Allergy and Infectious Diseases, in Hamilton, Montana, isolated corkscrew-shaped bacteria from ticks found in the areas where Lyme disease had occurred. These bacteria were subsequently named *Borrelia burgdorferi*.

The epidemiology of what we call Lyme disease has been traced to the late 1800s, however, and was first described in European literature in 1909 by Dr. Arvid Afzelius, who demonstrated to the Swedish Dermatological Society a migrating annular skin lesion, which he called "erythema migrans" (or EM rash), that had developed at the site of a bite by the sheep tick, *Ixodes ricinus*.

This syndrome and its attendant symptoms have always been referred to in European medical documentation as "Erythema chronicum migrans," or ECM, because of their long duration. It was only in the fall of 1992, when Dr. Burgdorfer, in an attempt to standardize descriptions for a medical profile on the disease, surveyed the international medical community that all parties agreed to accept the term "Lyme disease."

According to articles in the *Washington Post,* however, a genetic analysis of rodent pelts that have been stored in museums since the late 1800s revealed that much of the material gathered tested positive for the Lyme bacteria. And independent researchers have been gathering evidence suggesting that infected ticks might have even arrived in New York Harbor on the pelts of imported Russian furs.

More disturbing is the research and records of John Loftus—who, under President Jimmy Carter, served as a member of the newly formed Office of Special Investigations. In his book, *The Belarus Secret: The Nazi Question in America,* Loftus, an attorney given the highest security clearances available, recounts how he was instructed to go through long-buried and confidential war records, and how he came across documents of Nazi germ-warfare scientists who experimented with infected ticks dropped from planes to spread diseases.

The Centers for Disease Control (CDC), which is responsible for tracking infectious illness in the United States, has set specific surveillance criteria for reporting purposes that have both allowed public health agencies to follow the spread of the disease and provided grounds for confusion regarding diagnosis (see chapter 6). At the time of this writing, Lyme disease is considered endemic—or regularly occurring—in Connecticut, Rhode Island, New Jersey, New York, Delaware, Pennsylvania, Massachusetts, Maryland, Wisconsin, Minnesota, New Hampshire, and Vermont. These states accounted for 95 percent of the nationally reported cases in 2002. In addition, as both the public and physicians became educated in recognizing the signs and symptoms of Lyme disease, a number of other states have seen a huge increase in reported cases, including Missouri, Florida, Virginia, North Carolina, Texas, California, Ohio, and Illinois.

In 2002, the CDC recorded 23,764 Lyme disease cases that fit its strict criteria—a "record number," according to officials. But—and this is a big "but"—the CDC is also now clear that this number represents only 5 to 10 percent of the actual cases of Lyme, due to nonreporting on the part of the physicians and states, as well as the stringent reporting criteria, which fit less than 40 percent of true Lyme cases overall. In some hyperendemic areas, certain communities report that up to 20 percent of the population is infected. Thus, in actuality, the number of Lyme cases for 2002 may be as high as 250,000, and there are many physicians who maintain the actual numbers are double that.

These numbers concern not only health officials in the United States but those in the international medical community as well. The spread of Lyme disease has gained epidemic proportions throughout Canada, where Health Canada's Laboratory Centre for Disease Control reports that *Borrelia*-infected black-legged ticks have been found in every province between Manitoba and Newfoundland and are endemic at Long Point and Point Pelee on Lake Erie. Its cousin, the western black-legged tick is endemic in the Fraser River delta, the Gulf Islands, and Vancouver Island.

In Europe, information from the World Health Organization and several studies being conducted in Sweden shows that the extent of Lyme infection is startling, particularly considering that few countries have made Lyme a compulsorily notifiable disease. It is considered endemic in Germany (where it is estimated that 10 to 15 percent of the entire population is infected), Austria, France, Sweden, the Czech Republic, Bulgaria, and Slovenia in addition to portions of China, Japan, Australia, the United Kingdom, twenty-seven Russian territories, and numerous other European countries.

The big questions regarding the spread of Lyme are how and why and what the government plans to do regarding research funding for a cure.

VECTORS AND HOSTS

In the United States, Lyme disease has been documented as being spread by the *Ixodes* tick. In the North and Southeast it is commonly the *Ixodes scapularis* (formerly called *Ixodes dammini*), and in the West the *Ixodes pacificus*. In addition, it has now been confirmed that infection is also transmitted by the Lone

Star tick (*Amblyomma americanum*) in the midwestern and western states, and there is some reporting of infection from the American dog tick (*Dermacentor variabilis*).

In Europe and Asia the predominant vectors, or carriers, of Lyme disease are *Ixodes ricinus* and *Ixodes persulcatus*. There is some controversy both in Europe and in the United States as to whether Lyme is also passed on by other biting insects—such as the mosquito, flea, and horsefly—and some documented cases of this do exist.

These vectors feed on dozens of mammals, birds, and reptiles, which may then serve as reservoirs to infect other ticks. During the tick's three-stage life cycle, it passes from larva to nymph (80 percent of human Lyme disease cases are acquired during this stage) to adult (accounting for the remaining 20 percent). The size of the tick is approximately the size of the period at the end of this sentence.

Despite the fact that the tick must be connected to a human for at least four to twenty-four hours in order to spread infection, its size, coupled with the fact that it injects an anesthetic into the human skin upon both puncturing and withdrawing, makes it difficult to detect easily.

Although deer and the white-footed mouse have carried the brunt of the blame for spreading the infected ticks, their limited geographic ranges could not account for the rapid spread of the disease. Researchers now agree that infected ticks are hitching rides on ninety-nine different species of migrating birds—and, in fact, tick infestations peak during autumn migration, when an estimated ten billion birds travel up to seven thousand kilometers from summer breeding grounds to winter quarters. During their travels, land birds frequently stop to rest and eat, and they may acquire and pass infected ticks along the way.

In addition, other hosts for infected ticks include more than thirty species of small mammals, including rabbits, voles, chipmunks, and even domestic pets who spend a significant portion of their day out-of-doors. In Europe, additional hosts have included foxes and hedgehogs. And not only can you contract

Lyme disease from the infected tick, the disease has been documented in those exposed to the urine or blood of infected animals.

Some researchers maintain that Lyme disease is not necessarily spreading; they say that there is just a greater awareness of it, which has, in turn, caused increasing hysteria, rather than increasing case numbers. This criticism is just wishful thinking. Recent epidemiologic studies find that not only is the tick vector spreading and the percentage of infected ticks increasing, but that such environmental changes as global warming, resulting in warmer winters, have contributed to the lengthened span of the ticks' activity. And despite the indisputable fact that the summer months are prime Lyme season, infection can occur during virtually any month of the year—depending upon one's level of outdoor activity, one's profession, the weather, the geographic location, vacation trips, and whether infected ticks ride into the house on stray mammals (such as mice) seeking warmth during winter months.

Since, at the present time, the most effective weapons against Lyme disease are education and prevention, public health officials, environmentalists, and animal rights advocates are being called upon to assess the efficacy of insecticides and control of the deer population (see chapter 20).

OTHER MEANS OF TRANSMISSION

There is much controversy over the possibility of transmission of Lyme disease by means other than a tick bite. Since the Lyme spirochete, in later stages, has been isolated from various body fluids, there is much discussion regarding the passing of the Lyme infection through blood transfusions, sexual relations, and breast milk.

The Red Cross will not allow anyone who has had an active Lyme disease infection during the preceding year to be a blood donor. Various research studies have shown that the spirochete can live under blood bank conditions for up to several months. In addition, there is a small number of documented cases where a person apparently has been infected through a blood transfusion.

A growing number of doctors agree that not only can Lyme disease be transmitted through the placenta—Dr. Charles Ray Jones, a New Haven pediatrician, says, "Of the more than five thousand children I've treated with Lyme, two hundred forty have been born with the disease"—but it can also be passed to an infant through breast milk. Again, continuing studies have isolated the spirochete from breast milk and seem to support this position.

One of the more controversial theories is that Lyme can also be transmitted sexually. Although this has not been proven at this time, a number of reputable clinicians maintain that, due to the spirochete's presence in body fluids, the amount of fluid ejaculated during sexual relations would be enough to transmit the spirochete from the male to the female. Like syphilis, Lyme disease is caused by a spirochete. No one disputes that syphilis can be sexually transmitted, so the thinking in many circles is that the *Borrelia* spirochete behaves much the same way. A number of cases of husband/wife infection have been documented, but further studies have to be undertaken before infection through sexual transmission is proven with any certainty. This is the focus of a new study and a pending paper by Dr. Steven Phillips, a Wilton, Connecticut, physician and researcher whose last seven-year project resulted in a promising test for detecting spirochetes in an infected patient's blood.

THE CONTROVERSIES AND COSTS

There is no honor in being at the cutting edge of an epidemic.
—Dr. Richard Goldman, Gainesville, Florida, Lyme support group leader

Darlene is sure she contracted Lyme disease when she was on vacation with her family the year before she entered college. She spent the next four years passing through the revolving door of medical tests, drugs, and increasing symptoms. Her mood swings, fatigue, and varying symptoms cost her a marriage, a job in a brokerage house, and several family relationships. After a suicide attempt, she was assigned to a northeastern psychiatric hospital. When one of the physicians in the hospital, who had been researching Lyme and the illnesses it imitates, initiated Lyme tests for the patients, he was shocked to find that nearly 40 percent of those residing in the psychiatric hospital tested positive. Now, at thirty-four, after six months on intravenous antibiotics, Darlene is just beginning to pick up the life she left behind at eighteen.

In today's society, when one feels ill, the course of action is usually quite simple. Depending upon the nature of the symptoms, one might visit a specialist or an internist, who will record the complaints, mentally process the information, issue a diagnosis, and prescribe either a pharmacological remedy or/and a change of habit.

In those cases where symptoms may suggest two or three alternatives, or differential diagnoses, corroborating tests are usually ordered to confirm one or the other, and then a prescription is written. Within a given time period, unless the illness requires surgery or falls into one of the arenas involving AIDS, cancer, or chronic illness, the patient is cured and continues life as before.

Not only have we come to embrace this "cookbook" approach to medical care, doctors themselves are trained to promote it.

Then came Lyme disease. Because of its varied symptoms (many of which are subjective and immeasurable), its varied intensities, its varied stages of development, its ability to masquerade as a number of other illnesses, and the lack of reliable testing procedures for it, Lyme disease has challenged traditional medical practices, polarized the medical community, and raised serious questions regarding health care costs, insurance coverage, and medical malpractice.

It cannot be emphasized enough that Lyme disease, if diagnosed early and treated immediately (defined as within the first six weeks following a tick bite), can usually be resolved without further complications. The problems arise from the following facts:

- More than half of Lyme victims do not remember being bitten by a tick (a tick bite does not hurt due to the anesthetic the tick injects upon both puncturing and withdrawing).
- More than 60 percent of victims do not exhibit a telltale rash (one of the CDC's reportorial requirements—and this includes not just a "classic" bull's-eye rash but ten documented variations).
- The time lapse between the tick bite and emergence of symptoms can be weeks to months due to the spirochete's slow replication and ability to lie dormant in the human cell, and this can lead to chronic infection.
- Generally accepted testing procedures have had only a 30 to 40 percent reliability rate, at best.
- Too many physicians are ignorant of the disease's complexities at this time.
- Without definitive tests, many physicians have been reluctant to make a diagnosis and begin treatment due to possible malpractice suits.
- Treatment is also a source of disagreement since Lyme does not fit normal patterns of infectious disease containment.

The innate structure of the medical community also lends itself to controversy. There is a traditional dichotomy between basic research (sometimes called "academic" research) and clinical practice.

The researcher wants to control all the variables (as in double-blind studies); therefore subjects are selected, treated, and evaluated uniformly so that scientific principles can be standardized and scientific outcomes can be replicated. The clinician, the "doctor in the trenches" who daily deals closely with suffering people, wants the freedom to treat each patient as an individual, not as a research subject, thus allowing for the very real variations that exist in diagnosis, treatment, and patient response.

Normally, a partnership that meets both sets of needs is forged between the two groups for the overall benefit of science and the patient. But the Lyme spirochete and ensuing infection are proving to be outside the bounds of what has been considered "normal." Therefore, the approach to the disease is going through tremendous "growing pains" even in the heat of battle, complete with verbal missiles launched by both camps of doctors, each with the intention of discrediting the other. Until more time has passed, more documentation has been accepted, more physicians have been educated, more reliable tests have been developed, and more curative antibiotics have been discovered, there will be a difference of opinion and approach.

The media, however well-meaning, have also contributed to the controversy. Whether it is due to lack of space, lack of access to information, or lack of interest in accurately portraying this complex and contradictory medical phenomenon, media coverage has varied from hysterical to myopic to outright denial of the problem.

For example, in the book *Disease Mongers,* author Lynn Payer wrote from a generally confrontational bias against the bombardment of the population by those with a medical agenda to fulfill. She alluded to hysteria over reported Lyme cases and Americans' fear of germs and chose to quote only those few select medical experts who admit to espousing the most conservative (academic) stand regarding Lyme disease despite published documentation to the contrary. This type of one-sided reporting is just as damaging to the education of the public and recognition of a potential health hazard as the denial of the disease's existence and lack of *any* education. Lyme disease, as both researchers and the public are discovering, is not so easily dispensed with in a few simplistic pages.

Finally, there are those self-interested people who are simply out to make a buck off a new phenomenon and who see a new disease as an opportunity for personal and financial advancement. These opportunists can set back the acceptance of well-grounded research and treatment recommendations with tainted practices and attitudes.

But whichever controversy is strongest at the moment, the one who pays the cost is the Lyme disease patient and his or her family, because this is a disease that affects more than just the victim.

And the longer the time between tick bite and diagnosis and treatment, the more serious the implications and the higher the costs.

THE APPARENT COSTS

I scanned my checkbook (can't have a test without a check!) and
was able to add up an interesting history before Katie was diagnosed. She saw ten M.D.'s (that we recall) and had three upper
endoscopies, one colonoscopy, one lumbar puncture, three upper GI
series, one ultrasound, one CAT scan, one MRI, two small bowel
series, and blood work done over thirty times (only one was a Lyme
titer that I know of). Isn't it unbelievable what our kids have had to
endure? The worst part was the lack of understanding and disbelief
among the doctors and even our own family!

—Liz, registered nurse and mother of teenage Lyme victim,
Westchester County, New York

In a one-year study conducted jointly by the Society of Actuaries
and the Lyme Disease Foundation in 1991 and revised in 1993, the
costs of Lyme disease to society were explored. Of the 573 cases
originally submitted, the study limited itself to the 503 that reported
a documented diagnosis of Lyme disease by a physician.

The study was spearheaded by Dr. Irwin Vanderhoof, an econ-
omist and retired adjunct professor at New York University's
Stern School of Business, and its results included the following:

- The average number of doctors seen prior to diagnosis was 5.
- A family practitioner diagnosed 146 of the cases; an internist, 96;
  infectious disease specialist, 85; rheumatologist, 71; neurologist,
  70; and other specialists, 69.
- The average lost income before diagnosis was $7,877.
- The average total of medical bills prior to diagnosis was $14,797.
- The average lost income after diagnosis was $6,454.
- The average total of medical bills after diagnosis was $32,560.
- This all came to a grand total of $61,688.

▪ Further analysis of the data, based on the number of months between the contraction of the disease and its diagnosis, emphasizes the importance of early diagnosis and treatment:

Less than six months until diagnosis—$34,557 average total cost

Seven to twelve months—$68,233 average total cost

Over twelve months—$91,519 average total cost

An examination of individual records determined that 20 percent of the cases—those reporting the largest amounts of cost—represented 80 percent of the total costs. "This is the same relationship we would expect for medical claims in general and those reported to insurance companies," said Dr. Vanderhoof. "The distribution of cost amounts then provides additional credibility to the data. These largest-cost cases averaged thirty-one months from infection to diagnosis and were mostly cases that had some course of treatment with intravenous antibiotics. The average cost reported by these patients was almost $250,000 per case."

This 1993 study determined that Lyme disease was costing approximately $1 billion per year. Just three years later, another cost analysis, published by the Lewin Group of Mechelen, Belgium, in conjunction with MEDTAP International in Bethesda, Maryland, noted that the direct and indirect cost of Lyme disease to patients, the economy, and society, had skyrocketed to $2.5 billion.

Of course, accurate cost determination also goes back to accurate reporting, which concerns the CDC (see chapter 7). Dr. David Dennis, chief of the CDC's Bacterial Zoonoses Branch and director of its Lyme Disease Program, initiated a survey of fifty-two families throughout five school districts in hyperendemic New York State in cooperation with the Wharton School of Business to further determine the costs of Lyme.

In addition to the dollar figures, which are consistent with those found by Dr. Vanderhoof, the CDC study also found that among children with Lyme:

- 140 school days were lost, with an average of 98 days of home instruction needed
- 80 percent experienced a drop in grades
- 100 percent had to stop normal social activities
- 80 percent experienced a significant decrease in friendships and other social relationships
- Schools spent $130,000 providing at-home tutoring programs for incapacitated kids
- Total cost per child in the survey, including parents' lost time from work, tests, and treatment, came to $100,000

"Congress allocated $5.4 million for the entire Lyme disease project for 1992–93," said Dennis, "and the actual costs were around $5.2 million for just fifty-two kids. You can see what we're fighting here." In 2004 dollars, the numbers only look worse.

In the employment sector, the costs are also beginning to mount. In those areas where Lyme disease is considered endemic, major employers are not only straining to cover the costs of diagnostic testing and treatment through company benefits programs, but those such as Johnson & Johnson, which self-insures employees, are setting limits as to how much they will pay out.

The 3M Company in Minnesota took a leadership role in educating its population on Lyme by sponsoring a leave of absence for one of its afflicted scientists, Jo Ann Heltzel, with the assignment of researching and teaching the 3M community and its vast environs about the disease—a mission that Heltzel continues.

But aside from the mounting financial costs, the human costs in terms of both adults and children operating at diminished capacity cannot be so easily quantified, and the costs of suffering cannot be translated into dollars.

THE HIDDEN COSTS

At first glance, Sam, a forty-nine-year-old architectural designer, looks like a stereotypical professor or author. Bearded and of robust build, he lived an outdoor lifestyle on Nantucket with his wife and four children. He traces his Lyme disease to a hike he took in 1987. Through a year of increasing symptoms, beginning with a burning sensation on the bottoms of his feet and progressing to the eventual loss of the use of his legs, he found himself bedridden and dependent, and his symptoms viewed with skepticism. Five years later, he can no longer work at his profession, is divorced, lives in his parents' home, and struggles to simply rise from a chair and move across the room.

"I'm a stubborn Italian and I know I'm going to beat this," he says, "but this disease has cost me in ways you can't even imagine. Your self-esteem drops, you begin to doubt your own sanity, and then you start building walls between you and those around you because they just can't understand what's going on inside. I've always been a positive individual, gregarious, anti-chemical, anti-drug, and now my life has shrunk to just getting through the day. I know what will exacerbate the symptoms, but the limits change each day. What really hurts is what it did to my family," he says softly, eyes filling. "I can't blame my wife. I went through incredible mood swings, hostility, I didn't know what was happening to my body—and since nobody else knew either, no one could tell me, 'Hey, this is part of the disease and you'll get on top of it.' My kids are growing up and I can't be there for them like I'd like to be. I try, but some days are just a struggle to survive the pain. We have to educate not just the people, but the doctors as well. It's better to overdramatize maybe, and save one, than lose many because, man, you lose a whole family—not just a Lyme victim."

This story is echoed across the country. Active and upbeat people lose the capacity to perform their jobs; athletes lose their ability to play sports for recreation or profession; the emotional turmoil within family life roils to the point of divorce or separation as the Lyme victim—and in many families, more than one person is afflicted—stresses the climate of a household with constant symptoms, financial demands, and psychological changes (see chapter 6) that boomerang throughout both immediate family and extended relationships.

Because Lyme symptoms can include confusion, short-term memory loss, and disorientation, Lyme victims report withdrawal from not only social situations but also from driving automobiles, for fear of accidents, and from professional situations that might require them to speak before groups or take responsibility for others.

But the losses are even more insidious than that. Since recent studies show that 50 percent of Lyme victims are under the age of twelve, late diagnosis and treatment can result in a potential loss of thinkers, leaders, athletes, dancers, artists, and service providers. In short, the disease is invading the fabric of America's future.

The U.S. Department of Education created the Individualized Education Program (IEP) under the Individuals with Disabilities Education Act (1997) that will ensure specially designed instruction for each student with a documented disability (see chapter 9). It mandates that those children who are too sick to attend school, or can only attend school part-time, are entitled to a program of instruction, tutoring, and help based upon their own unique needs. This has been one of the cornerstones of keeping children with Lyme engaged in the educational process, even with a diminished capacity.

Even the conservative Educational Testing Service in Princeton, New Jersey, which has responsibility for the administering and grading of the SAT, has recognized the effect of Lyme disease on teenagers by implementing a special untimed test for those who can document the illness through a physician. And university admissions offices are becoming increasingly aware of the drop in performance during the high school years caused by Lyme and are accepting students who, again, provide adequate documentation.

Dr. Joseph Burrascano of Long Island, New York, is a nationally recognized Lyme researcher and clinician who contracted the disease when he was in his teens. He says that Lyme disease lowers one's level of performance and expectations. "Most of the time I felt lousy and I was sleeping sixteen hours a day, but that was normal for me. I didn't realize that other people didn't feel that way."

Lyme disease is changing the way many Americans are spending their leisure time. This includes eliminating nature walks and picnics, not playing in or raking fall leaves, and avoiding contact with certain family pets like dogs and cats in endemic areas. Schools are eliminating recreational and natural-science field trips and there are reports of summer camps closing in endemic areas.

Another real factor in Lyme disease is fear. Some say this is related to modern man's primal fear of the wilderness. But others contend that it is more anxiety and frustration at being attacked in one's own home, or "castle." Dr. Len Sigal, chief of rheumatology and director of the Lyme Disease Unit at Robert Wood Johnson Medical Center in New Brunswick, New Jersey, who cautions against the possible hysteria of seeing Lyme under every leaf, nevertheless understands the public's anxiety. "I moved out of the city so my children can grow up not getting mugged and breathing clean air. Now there's a silent and unseen danger lurking right out in our back yards. This is frustrating."

My grandmother, who seemingly had an adage for everything, loved to repeat that favorite "If you have your health, you have everything." For growing numbers of Lyme disease patients, the "everything" is elusive, resulting in the mental jump to "I have nothing." This is not true. These people have a will to survive, to fight, and to reclaim the good health they wistfully remember. The irony of Lyme disease is that anyone else fighting for health finds a pyramid of support, beginning with physicians and followed by larger tiers of associations, friends, and family.

Lyme disease victims, however, often find themselves stranded on the peak of the pyramid all alone, fighting for credibility, treatment, and simple compassion. Since the symptoms and signs are so varied and often transient, the patient needs to be vigilant in noticing and reporting these bodily and personality changes, and then in seeking the right doctor to put them all together.

2.

Recognizing Symptoms and Seeking Help

When my son was becoming progressively more ill, prior to his Lyme diagnosis, the wide variety of his symptoms seemed staggering; his complaints were constant and every system of his body was involved. In fact, it got to the point where I wondered if he could possibly be making them up, and he wondered if he should even tell me everything that was going on.

As both his body and his personality continued a marked deterioration, however, it became apparent that something serious was definitely wrong. It wasn't until a good friend, who had traveled a similar road the prior year with her daughter, handed me some information on Lyme disease that I began to put the myriad symptoms into a definable context. The turning point was Dr. Burrascano's page of Lyme disease symptoms. In reading this and checking off what Chris had experienced, I realized that this child had thirty out of the forty symptoms listed! He was not a hypochondriac or going crazy, although he was sure he was headed in that direction.

That was twelve years ago. At that time, doctors dealing with Lyme disease divided it into early and late stages, depending upon the various manifestations of the infection. Since that time it has further been divided into four stages, as doctors and researchers gradually learn more and narrow down the disease's progress. But the doctors emphasize that these stages can overlap—due to individual body chemistry, one person can go from early localized (which is simply defined as evidence of EM rash) to late disseminated (where the infection has spread throughout many body systems) or even to chronic within months, while another will take months just to go from early localized to early disseminated.

For this reason, and for clarity's sake, I am going to ignore the stage breakdown at this time and simply present symptoms as they are known today. We will deal with stages in chapter 14.

In an attempt to document as complete a list of symptoms as possible, Kathy Cavert, a registered nurse from Independence, Missouri, editor of *LymeAid* and founder of the Midwest Lyme Disease Association, composed a questionnaire and distributed it to more than one thousand Lyme disease patients. In presenting the following list of symptoms, I have combined Dr. Burrascano's updated list with the format and additions of Cavert's.

LYME DISEASE SYMPTOMS

As part of your current illness, have you had any of the following?

▪ The Tick Bite

1. Tick bite (deer, dog, or other)	Yes	No
2. Rash at site of bite	Yes	No
3. Rashes on other parts of your body	Yes	No
4. Rash basically circular and spreading out	Yes	No
5. Raised rash, disappearing and returning	Yes	No

▪ Head, Face, Neck

6. Unexplained hair loss	Yes	No
7. Headache, mild or severe	Yes	No
8. Twitching of facial or other muscles	Yes	No
9. Facial paralysis (Bell's palsy)	Yes	No
10. Tingling of nose, cheek, or face	Yes	No
11. Stiff or painful neck, creaks and cracks	Yes	No
12. Jaw pain or stiffness	Yes	No
13. Sore throat	Yes	No

■ Eyes/Vision

    14. Double or blurry vision   Yes No

    15. Increased floating spots   Yes No

    16. Pain in eyes, or swelling around eyes   Yes No

    17. Oversensitivity to light   Yes No

    18. Flashing lights   Yes No

■ Ears/Hearing

    19. Decreased hearing in one or both ears   Yes No

    20. Buzzing in ears   Yes No

    21. Pain in ears, oversensitivity to sound   Yes No

    22. Ringing in one or both ears   Yes No

■ Digestive and Excretory Systems

    23. Diarrhea   Yes No

    24. Constipation   Yes No

    25. Irritable bladder (trouble starting, stopping)   Yes No

    26. Upset stomach (nausea or pain)   Yes No

■ Musculoskeletal System

    27. Joint pain or swelling   Yes No

    28. Stiffness of joints, back, neck   Yes No

    29. Muscle pain or cramps   Yes No

■ Respiratory and Circulatory Systems

    30. Shortness of breath, cough   Yes No

    31. Chest pain or rib soreness   Yes No

    32. Night sweats or unexplained chills   Yes No

    33. Heart palpitations or extra beats   Yes No

    34. Heart blockage   Yes No

■ Neurologic System

35. Tremors or unexplained shaking   Yes   No
36. Burning or stabbing sensations in the body   Yes   No
37. Weakness or partial paralysis   Yes   No
38. Pressure in head   Yes   No
39. Numbness in body, tingling, pinpricks   Yes   No
40. Poor balance, dizziness, difficulty walking
41. Increased motion sickness   Yes   No
42. Lightheadedness, wooziness   Yes   No

■ Psychological Well-being

43. Mood swings, irritability   Yes   No
44. Unusual depression   Yes   No
45. Disorientation (getting or feeling lost)   Yes   No
46. Feeling as if you are losing your mind   Yes   No
47. Overemotional reactions, crying easily   Yes   No
48. Too much sleep, or insomnia   Yes   No
49. Difficulty falling or staying asleep   Yes   No

■ Mental Capacity

50. Memory loss (short or long term)   Yes   No
51. Confusion, difficulty in thinking   Yes   No
52. Difficulty with concentration or reading   Yes   No
53. Going to the wrong place   Yes   No
54. Speech difficulty (slurred or slow)   Yes   No
55. Stammering speech   Yes   No
56. Forgetting how to perform simple tasks   Yes   No

■ Reproduction and Sexuality

57. Loss of sex drive   Yes   No
58. Sexual dysfunction   Yes   No
    Females only:

59. Unexplained menstrual pain, irregularity   Yes   No
60. Unexplained breast pain, discharge   Yes   No
    Males only:
61. Testicular or pelvic pain   Yes   No

■ General Well-being

62. Unexplained weight gain, loss   Yes   No
63. Extreme fatigue   Yes   No
64. Swollen glands   Yes   No
65. Unexplained fevers (high- or low-grade)   Yes   No
66. Continual infections (sinus, kidney, eye, etc.)   Yes   No
67. Symptoms seem to change, come and go   Yes   No
68. Pain migrates (moves) to different body parts   Yes   No
69. Early on, experienced a "flu-like" illness,   Yes   No
    after which you have not since felt well

As you can see, this is a daunting list of possible symptoms, but answering yes to many in various systemic categories should put both you and your doctor on the alert to consider Lyme disease.

As many doctors who treat Lyme patients say, at one time or another most of us will experience illness in one of our body's systems. If a person is unlucky, he or she can have two major systems involved. But when you begin having problems with multiple systems in the body, that is a red flag to consider a multisystemic infection like Lyme disease. This suspicion should be particularly warranted if you live in an area where Lyme is endemic.

One of the more frightening aspects of Lyme is that, unlike other purely systemic illnesses, it attacks not only the physical well-being of a person but the emotional and psychological components as well. Primary among these symptoms are the mood swings, memory loss, and confusion that Lyme sufferers experience.

The late Dr. John Bleiweiss of Trenton, New Jersey, who suffered from Lyme himself and dedicated the last ten years of his life to pioneering combination treatments and fighting for the rights of Lyme patients, always bristled at those doctors who dismissed Lyme as a minor irritation.

"This is the kind of disease which, if not recognized and treated promptly and completely, can affect the future of our country," said Bleiweiss. "I have seen active, outgoing people wind up in wheelchairs without the proper treatment. Nearly all patients complain of 'foggy brain' or 'Lyme fog,' forgetfulness, anxiety, and confusion or disorientation when attempting intellectual tasks.

"Short-term memory impairment causes patients to forget why they entered a room; forget the previous sentence or paragraph while reading; forget dates, schedules, where objects were placed, and even the names of family members. A mother with Lyme left her infant and baby carriage in my parking lot and went home. One patient wandered around the room looking for the pencil that was clenched in his teeth. One patient drove to Philadelphia by mistake instead of Princeton because both began with the letter P. In fact, patients can lose their way home, their way to work, or even the way to their classroom in a familiar school because they suddenly forget where they are," he said. "This is scary stuff. And when you think that more than fifty percent of those infected with Lyme disease are teenagers and kids, we're talking about a real impact on our future."

Since the symptoms of Lyme disease are so diverse and progressive, remembering them may be a chore in itself in presenting an accurate accounting to a doctor. The best method to employ is to write it all down.

KEEP A JOURNAL

Like most outdoors enthusiasts, Caitlin had her share of bug bites and rashes. An artist, aerobics instructor, and dedicated hiker and camper, she tried to live a healthful lifestyle and had little contact with doctors. Then she went hiking in the hills of upstate New York and her life changed irrevocably.

It began with a raised rash, warm to the touch. Since it was unusual, she made an appointment with her doctor. By the time of her appointment to see him two days later (rashes, she was told, are not priority cases) the rash had disappeared, so she canceled the appointment. Then came the headaches and stiff neck. Since she is active, she suspected that she had either overextended herself or slept wrong. When she began to lose the use of her right arm and hand, she went to see a neurologist, and one CAT scan, MRI, and spinal tap later, was told there was nothing wrong with her. The neurologist suggested that perhaps she just needed to take a break from her normal routine. Feeling confused, she ignored the sore throat, the change in bowel habits, and the increasing fatigue she felt. When she found that she was so dizzy she could barely walk, and her arm was so useless that she could not hold her toothbrush, she went to an internist, who ran another battery of tests, told her they were negative, and recommended she consider seeing a psychiatrist since, after all, she was twenty-eight years old and didn't have a steady boyfriend.

"I was so mad, that's when I began writing all the symptoms down," she said. "After a while, I began to think I was going crazy, since every day brought more aches and pains. I had to stop teaching aerobics, I could barely hold a paintbrush, and I was so depressed I didn't even want to be around people. When my mother called to ask how I was, I lied so I wouldn't sound like a hypochondriac and worry her."

Then she passed out in a grocery store and awoke in the hospital, connected to a heart monitor. A cardiologist told her that she had some extra heartbeats and she needed to take it easy and live a more healthful lifestyle. She never saw him after that. Six months later, Caitlin saw a television program on Lyme disease. A lot of what was being said began ringing bells in her head and she looked at her list of symptoms. She could track the deterioration of her health back to those fateful rashes. A visit to a local Lyme support group meeting put her in touch with a doctor who had experience in diagnosing and treating cases. Her symptom log assisted in his diagnosis.

Eighteen months after Caitlin saw the rash, she is on antibiotics and is beginning to experience a few pain-free days. "But my joints and back still hurt and I find I get lost sometimes. When that happens I just have to calm myself down and keep driving until something looks familiar again," she said with a sigh. "I have to think that someone will come up with a cure someday because there were so many things I wanted to do in life. Now I'm happy just to have a day where I don't drop things, don't have headaches, and can sleep through the night like a normal person."

Caitlin's case illustrates a couple of interesting points. First, by the time she could get a doctor's appointment, her rash was gone. Therefore, there was no documentation of the rash—the first criterion for reporting Lyme disease—by a physician. Second, Caitlin, accustomed to thinking in terms of medical specialties, in her attempt to get a diagnosis from her symptoms saw several different types of doctors, each of them only seeing what applied to his or her area of expertise. This is very common. It was only due to Caitlin's efficiency in writing down her symptoms that her physician was able to piece together a difficult diagnosis.

As information regarding Lyme disease spreads throughout the country, perhaps doctors will make room for patients who call complaining of suspicious rashes. Until then, I would encourage anyone with a suspicious rash to go to one of the fine walk-in emergency medical centers popping up across the country. No appointment is necessary, and if the rash turns out to be the hallmark of Lyme, you will have a doctor's confirmation of its presence.

Dr. Ernest Biczak trained in emergency medicine as preparation for opening his Immediate Medical Care Center in rural Chester, New Jersey. "Fifteen years ago when we opened, I thought we would be handling emergencies, but what we've turned into is a family practice." He chuckled. "This is what has been the greatest need in our area. And we've been seeing more Lyme rashes this year than ever before. Some days, we will get three in a single day. Other days, none. We have talked about bringing in a camera to photograph and document them and we may have to do that yet."

Since contracting Lyme disease begins with a very specific event—the bite of a tick—it presents a very definite onset of symptoms. Whether you remember a tick bite and rash, or fall into the 50 percent who don't, when experiencing vague, fluctuating, or increasingly disturbing symptoms it would be a good idea to take the time to write them all down in a time-line fashion to the best of your ability. Get a family member to help you, if you can't remember. Do not leave anything out—from mood swings to weakness in a particular extremity.

This symptom log or journal can be a simple listing of symptoms; you do not need to write long paragraphs. Some doctors advise their patients to include a "wellness indicator" as you are going through the testing and diagnosis process. This is simply a scale from 1 to 10, with 10 for feeling great and 1 for feeling the worst. Assign a number to each day to aid the documentation of progress or degeneration. This will assist doctors as they consider various diagnoses.

THE DIFFERENTIAL DIAGNOSES

Jo Ann was diagnosed as having multiple sclerosis. After six years of treatment for MS, with continual degeneration, she was tested for Lyme and found to have the disease. Treated with antibiotics, she began to recover her physical and mental abilities, her job performance, and her life. Today she is working to educate others regarding Lyme disease and includes the warning that it masquerades as many other illnesses, not the least of which is MS.

Twelve-year-old Dennis was told he had chronic mononucleosis and attention deficit disorder (ADD). As he deteriorated from a normal, active adolescent with hopes and dreams to sitting in a wheelchair and being assigned to a special education class, his parents struggled for help. He was finally tested for Lyme, in spite of opposition from his pediatrician. After nine months of therapy, Dennis is finally rejoining his classmates in thinking about high school next year and trying out for sports teams.

Beverly felt her life was over when her doctor told her she had lupus. It was only after two years of meticulous research on the part of her husband and a change of doctors that she was tested for Lyme disease. Since she lives in Texas, an area where Lyme disease supposedly does not exist, she travels to California for treatments. It is a small price to pay, she says, for feeling better and getting back her life.

Lyme disease is a clinical diagnosis and may become a diagnosis of exclusion. This means that, unless you exhibit a classic rash and test positive by blood, the physician will attempt to eliminate all other possible diseases before making the Lyme diagnosis. This is not unreasonable. Called the "Great Imitator," Lyme disease, because of its myriad symptoms, can mimic two hundred other illnesses. As a result, it can be missed by doctors who are not well acquainted with its pathology and progress.

There are several diseases that Lyme mimics most frequently, and, in discussing Lyme with your doctor, he may give you a "differential" or alternate diagnosis as you go through the testing process. These include babesiosis, a malaria-like infection; Rocky Mountain spotted fever; and Human Granulocytic Ehrlichiosis, often referred to as HGE. Ehrlichiosis made headlines as the "Lyme disease that kills" before researchers were able to isolate the bacteria. Because HGE is carried by the same ticks that carry Lyme, it is increasingly common for a victim to be infected with both diseases.

We will discuss this and several other tick-borne diseases that are complicating the Lyme diagnosis—and indeed, many Lyme patients' lives—in chapter 3.

Multiple sclerosis   A chronic, demyelinating central nervous system disease, similar to Lyme. Recent medical literature has drawn parallels between the two diseases in that magnetic resonance imaging (MRI) tests cannot distinguish between Lyme and MS; spirochetes have also been found in the spinal fluid and tissue samples of MS patients; and great clusters of MS victims have appeared in those areas of the United States and around the world where Lyme is now endemic. Some researchers are studying whether the Lyme spirochete, in fact, could be one of the causes of MS or if the Lyme spirochete produces an MS-like illness.

Fibromyalgia   An inflammation of the connective tissues of the body. It is a chronic pain syndrome characterized by diffuse muscle and joint pain; headache; abnormal spontaneous sensations such as burning, pricking, and numbness; sleep disturbances; and fatigue. Symmetric tender points are usually found in various locations over the neck, back, and extremities. Women are affected more frequently than men, with no apparent explanation.

While fibromyalgia was little known and poorly understood fifteen years ago, it is now more widely recognized but not understood much better. Many doctors feel that fibromyalgia is an indication of Lyme disease rather than a disease itself, and just as many will test for Lyme to eliminate it as a diagnosis. In one study of one hundred consecutive new patients seen at a Lyme disease referral center, 25 percent had fibromyalgia rather than chronic Lyme, but in approximately 70 percent of the cases, the fibromyalgia *followed* apparent Lyme disease, thus supporting the theory that fibromyalgia is caused by Lyme.

Systemic lupus   A disease characterized by inflammation in many different systems. Patients may have fatigue, anemia, fever, rashes, sun sensitivity, arthritis, pleurisy, hair loss, and nervous system disease. This disease, like Lyme, waxes and wanes in intensity, and its hallmark is a distinctive "butterfly" rash across the face.

Infectious mononucleosis   An acute infection caused by the Epstein-Barr virus. Symptoms include fever, sore throat, swollen glands, and fatigue. When confronted with confusing symptoms, some doctors have diagnosed chronic mono, but many more debate its existence, labeling it a "catchall" diagnosis.

Amyotrophic lateral sclerosis (ALS)   Also known as Lou Gehrig's disease, it affects the muscles in a single limb or all four limbs simultaneously and runs a course from two to seven years. A fatal disease, it usually strikes those in their fifties to seventies. Despite extensive research, the cause of ALS remains unknown at this time.

Chronic fatigue syndrome (CFS)   This disease, also referred to as the Yuppie disease, is caused by a virus and therefore does not respond to antibiotic treatment. Since severe fatigue—in fact, chronic fatigue—is a hallmark of Lyme disease, there are many doctors who insist that many Lyme patients are being misdiagnosed without being given a chance to be treated. Five million people have been diagnosed with CFS, yet the diagnosis is confusing, says Joe Burke, founder of the American Lyme Disease Alliance and formerly diagnosed with CFS. "A lot of the people who go to chronic fatigue support groups are also Lyme disease patients; many more exhibit classic Lyme symptoms but won't even seek a Lyme test or diagnosis because having CFS is a more comfortable plateau than looking further."

Alzheimer's disease   This most common of the progressive dementias affects both men and women. It primarily strikes the elderly and can exhibit many of the symptoms of Lyme, especially those of a cognitive nature; therefore a particular danger of misdiagnosis exists when dealing with senior citizens (see chapter 12).

Another roadblock to the accurate diagnosis of Lyme is the type of doctor you seek out. Because Lyme affects many systems of the body, a specialist for one system may not be able to look at the total picture of symptomology and make the diagnosis.

For example, the neurologist will consider the headaches but not the heart palpitations or joint pain. The rheumatologist will focus on the joint pain and the immune system but will probably pay little attention to the deterioration of your eyesight that is going on concurrently, referring you to an ophthalmologist . . . and so on.

Your primary line of attack should be an internist or family medicine practitioner, who should begin with a thorough patient history, some basic tests, and then coordinate with other specialists as needed. You need someone who can look at the overall picture and put the puzzle of Lyme disease together.

This, of course, assumes that the doctor you see is willing to work with you to find the right diagnosis. The key words here are "work with you."

THE VOLATILE DOCTOR-PATIENT RELATIONSHIP

When Lauren was five, she was diagnosed with Lyme disease after eleven months of misdiagnoses. Treated for three months, she seemed relieved of all symptoms and continued with life. When she was eight years old, her symptoms seemed to be returning. Back again were the joint pains, the headaches, and the stomachaches, plus—a new wrinkle—pain in her chest.

Her mother, taking her to a new pediatrician (her old one had retired), mentioned that Lauren had previously suffered from Lyme and had responded to treatment. In view of the medical literature indicating that the spirochete can lie dormant in the body for years and then flare up, she wanted the doctor to know her daughter's background. Since they live in one of the most highly endemic areas of Lyme disease in New Jersey, she felt this information would be pertinent in case the chest pains and other symptoms were part of the old disease rather than a new one.

"The doctor went crazy," said the stunned mother. "He actually screamed at me that Lyme disease was being blown out of proportion by hysterical women and disreputable doctors. He accused me of looking for Lyme under every symptom, and blasted me for mentioning the recent articles on Lyme, saying,

'And just where does one go to be an expert in Lyme disease, huh? Are there schools that teach Lyme disease?' He refused to examine my daughter that day—said he didn't have enough time because he had 'really sick patients to see' and that I could make another appointment if I felt it was really necessary.

"I can't believe he treated us that way. He refused to see a child who was complaining of chest pain and went nuts on me, all because I was trying to give him an accurate background to evaluate my daughter. Believe me, I am not a hysteric, but that doctor is also not a responsible physician! I wonder how many kids in this area are sick with Lyme because he refuses to even consider it when examining his patients!"

Approximately sixteen thousand new doctors graduate from this country's 128 medical schools each year. Somewhere between internship and residency, unfortunately, many new doctors tend to develop an arrogance that goes beyond the confidence one must have in order to make life-and-death decisions for another human being. While this arrogance is variously tolerated by baby boomers and expected by senior citizens, it can serve as an obstacle to good care.

Unfortunately, too, this arrogance is encouraged by the very people it can hurt. In this age of medical miracles, when we expect quick cures to difficult problems, the physician is trained to come up with those answers and cures. In fact, he is trained to come up with something—anything—when the patient asks a question; for to say, "I don't know" is viewed as the ultimate sin.

There is a lot that scientists, researchers, and doctors admit they don't know about Lyme disease. Worse yet, there is much that is known and ignored in medical teachings and practice. Those who make that admission and proceed from there are light-years ahead of those who deny the ubiquitous and diffuse nature of the illness because they are threatened by not having the answers.

There are two cardinal rules in coping with Lyme or suspected Lyme disease:

1. Do not accept ignorance or arrogance from your doctor.
2. Take an advocate with you to your medical appointments.

DO NOT ACCEPT IGNORANCE OR ARROGANCE FROM YOUR DOCTOR

When you take your car in for repair, you expect the mechanic to listen to your list of complaints, make his own observations, and then attempt to fix your car. If you get that car back, but it is still rattling at fifty miles per hour, you would probably return it to the mechanic and point out the problem. You would, rightly, expect him to work on it again to find out what the cause of the rattle could be.

If, however, the mechanic told you that the rattle was all in your head, belittled your intelligence, cross-examined you, and stated that if he said it was fixed, then it was fixed, would you go back to him? Of course not.

Yet many of us don't give our bodies and our health the same respect that we give our cars. The mechanic may know more about cars, but it does not follow that you cannot make valid observations.

By the same token, when confronted by a doctor who does not listen, will not take the time to ask questions of you, is threatened by your questions or information, and tells you that "she" is the doctor and "you" are the patient and therefore know little about medicine, you must fire her and search for a doctor who will work with you.

When seeking a physician, you need to do your homework. The following steps should be followed:

1. Call his/her office manager and ask how familiar the physician is with treating Lyme disease patients.

2. Inquire if the doctor has informational material to help in patient education.

3. If you decide to make an appointment, ask how much time is allotted to the first appointment. If the first appointment is less than thirty minutes (ideally, it should be an hour), request the additional time. If it is refused, look elsewhere.

Alfred Adler, often referred to as the father of individual (termed Adlerian) psychology, wrote about the arrogance of doctors back in the 1930s. He said: "To be a physician may mean many things. Not only may he wish to be a specialist . . . but he will show in his activities his own peculiar degree of interest in himself and interest in others. We shall see how far he trains himself to be of help to his fellows and how far he limits his helpfulness. He has made this his aim as a compensation for a specific feeling of inferiority; and we must be able to guess, from his expressions in his profession and elsewhere, the specific feeling for which he is compensating."

Any doctor who is threatened by a reasonably questioning patient is not someone you can trust to work with you.

It is equally unproductive, however, for a patient to walk into a doctor's office, present a list of symptoms and a diagnosis, and demand therapy of a specific sort. Confronted with that kind of patient, more often than not, a doctor could reasonably say, "Why do you need me if you have all the answers?"

TAKE AN ADVOCATE

Anyone who has received either shocking or complicated medical information knows that the mind tends to block the flow of information with emotional linebackers. Afterward, you might wonder, "What did the doctor say again?"

Since short-term memory loss, confusion, and fatigue are definite hallmarks of Lyme, it is a particular advantage to have a relative or other advocate present to absorb the doctor's spoken information, assist in remembering symptoms and events, and help with recommended tests or therapies.

Most children have a built-in advocate in Mom or Dad—whoever is the primary parent taking them through the sick-to-well process. But sick adults—particularly those who suspect Lyme—need an advocate as well.

Even in the best of circumstances, when one is ill it is difficult to remember all that the doctor has said and recommended. A discussion of Lyme disease can provoke anxiety that causes the patient's memory to go blank, and it helps to have another pair of eyes and ears and another brain to absorb, remember, and ask the right questions.

Remember that a pencil and paper are your lifeline. Take notes! You should arrive for your first visit prepared with notes about your symptoms, a symptoms time line, and a list of medications taken. You or your advocate must take note of the doctor's recommendations and treatment plan. This caring team approach includes patient, doctor, and family in the treatment process.

As we are confronted with a variety of new drug-resistant bacterias, and increasingly complex diseases and lifestyles, a new type of doctor-patient relationship must be forged: a partnership whereby the doctor and the patient (the medical consumer) work together to seek resolution of a medical problem. We must work toward a "therapeutic alliance."

But first, let's deal with some of the major complications to a simple Lyme diagnosis.

3.

Co-infections Mean Complications

As if it weren't difficult enough to nail down the sometimes elusive diagnosis of Lyme disease, the past six years have brought about the recognition that another ten illnesses are also transmitted to humans by the very same ticks that carry the Lyme spirochete and, in fact, may be transmitted at the same time. These include:

Babesiosis A malaria-like infection caused by piroplasms including *Babesia* protozoa. To complicate things further, one type of piroplasm in the eastern United States (*Babesia microti*) and a different species in the Midwest and West (MO-1 and WA-1) can be transmitted by black-legged ticks and the *Ixodes scapularis*. More than fifty cases of babesiosis acquired through blood transfusions have also been reported to the CDC. Babesiosis is on the rise and endemic in many of the same geographic areas as Lyme. Symptoms include fever, day and night sweats, fatigue, anemia, headache, chills, and muscle pain. Babesiosis may be self-limited in persons with an intact immune system but can be more serious, and even deadly, in the elderly and those who are immune-compromised or have had their spleens removed. It can be detected by a Giemsa-stain blood smear antibody test, a Bm-PCR, or an RNA-based test called the Flourescent In situ Hybridization, available through labs such as IGeneX in Palo Alto, California. If babesiosis is present, it fluoresces green on the blood smear. As with Lyme disease, the Red Cross will not accept blood from anyone who has been infected with babesiosis since it can be transmitted through the blood supply. It is possible that babesiosis can survive antiparasitic therapy and result in chronic, nonspecific multisystem symptoms, which can be difficult to distinguish from symptoms of organic Lyme disease.

Human Granulocytic Ehrlichiosis   Often referred to as ehrlichia, ehrlichiosis made headlines as Lyme "the disease that kills" before researchers were able to isolate the bacteria that invade and destroy white blood cells. Carried by the same ticks as Lyme, ehrlichiosis is becoming increasingly common (people can be infected with both Lyme and ehrlichiosis). Symptoms are similar to Lyme disease except that they are more severe and abrupt. Painful muscle aches, severe headaches, high fever, chills, sudden loss of appetite, a sudden drop in white blood cell and platelet counts, and elevated liver function could indicate ehrlichiosis, which responds to treatment with doxycycline and other tetracycline antibiotics. It does not respond, however, to amoxicillin and other antibiotics used to treat Lyme, which makes the proper diagnosis of this disease imperative.

The prevalence of Lyme-infected ticks co-infected with either or both babesiosis and ehrlichiosis has been the subject of recent studies and published papers. In those studies, researchers found that approximately 25 percent of the ticks in certain Lyme-endemic areas of New Jersey and New York infected with B. *burgdorferi* were also infected with ehrlichiosis and/or B. *microti*.

Bartonella   Often referred to as "cat scratch fever." Approximately 22,000 cases are reported each year, primarily transmitted through the bite or scratch of a cat or bite of a cat flea, although some doctors are reporting bartonella as present in Lyme patients as well since bartonella is also transmissible by tick bite. Symptoms include papules at the site of the bite, swollen lymph nodes, muscle aches, fever, and fatigue. In a small percentage of patients, infection can spread through the body, sometimes to the central nervous system. Laboratory confirmation can be obtained by indirect fluorescent antibody (IFA) testing for bartonella.

Relapsing Fever   A multisystem disease caused by three other *Borrelia* spirochetes that are different from *B. burgdorferi*. It occurs primarily, but not exclusively, in the western United States and is particularly virulent—the spirochetes can be transmitted within minutes, rather than hours. Symptoms include headache, chills, repeated bouts of high fever, and joint pain lasting two days to a week, followed by no pain and fever, followed by a relapse. Blood tests can detect the bacterium during fever episodes.

Rocky Mountain Spotted Fever   First recognized in 1896 in the Snake River Valley of Idaho, it was originally called "black measles" because of the characteristic rash. It is known to be spread by the American dog tick, Pacific Coast tick, and the Rocky Mountain wood tick; the Lone Star tick is under study as well. Symptoms include flu-like aches and pains, chills, confusion, headache, sensitivity to light, and high fever. The rash is distinguished by starting on the extremities and spreading to the trunk of the body. By the 1900s, the disease was so widespread and dreaded that the Rocky Mountain Laboratories in Hamilton, Montana, was established to study it. Now under the umbrella of the National Institute of Allergy and Infectious Diseases (NIAID) of the National Institutes of Health, the researchers at Rocky Mountain Labs have been at the forefront of studying Lyme and other tick-borne infections.

While the researchers conduct tests and design studies, the doctors in the field are being forced to self-educate, assess patients, and develop clinical protocols to treat the thousands who may have been diagnosed with Lyme disease but, despite the doctors' best efforts, are not getting well.

One of the pioneers in the area of co-infections is Dr. Richard Horowitz of Hyde Park, New York, who is credited with being the first to document the co-infection of babesiosis in inland areas such as Dutchess County. Educated on two continents, vice president of the International Lyme and Associated Disease Society, author of nearly two dozen papers on Lyme and other tick-borne diseases, and on the faculty of Marist College, Horowitz lives and practices amid the lush foliage that comprises one of the most endemic areas of the country.

On the way to the Hudson Valley Healing Arts Center (HVHAC), established by Horowitz six years ago to integrate traditional medicine with nutrition, psychology, and adjunctive therapies such as acupuncture and meditation, you pass the multi-turreted buildings and manicured campus of the Culinary Institute of America (CIA) just north of Poughkeepsie on Route 9. In a modern, grayish green building that nearly blends into the surrounding trees, he handles a patient load of 5,000 to 6,000 men, women, and children who travel from all parts of the country when their own physicians hit a diagnostic wall.

There is a sense of quiet confidence and Zen-like calm in Horowitz's insistence that doctors who are treating Lyme patients need to consider and test for multiple co-infections, particularly when treatment doesn't seem to help. It is a confidence born of years of research, erroneous criticism for thinking outside the box, and finally, scientific validation.

"The role of co-infections at this point is huge," he says. "For many patients it is as important—if not more important—as Lyme disease. They will not get better until the co-infections are found and treated. Ticks are containing more than ten organisms at this point. You may have to combine antibiotic regimens because one drug alone may not be enough. You need to hit the Lyme and the co-infections simultaneously. The trick for me is a two-drug intracellular regimen of doxycycline and cipro. With these, I see significant improvement."

This multimodal approach includes administering two to three antibiotics at the same time, each designed to attack one or more element of the infections. Knowing that the Lyme spirochete alone has the ability to shield itself, hide intracellularly, and adopt a cystic form to evade antibiotics, it is important that the treating physician be cognizant not only of the most effective drug to reach the Lyme spirochete but of the most efficient antibiotics to attack the co-infections as well.

Horowitz's documentation of the babesiosis co-infection with Lyme, through laboratory results and successful patient treatment, has recently been hailed as a major breakthrough. It is, he says, just what physicians were meant to do.

"I look at this as a doctor and ask myself the question, 'What can I do to benefit society at the greatest level?' The highest good I can do is be in service to my community. It's important for doctors to put themselves in the patients' shoes.

"I've been studying with a spiritual teacher for twenty-two years, and this way of thinking is called 'exchanging yourself for others.' You do what you would want done for yourself—which means you don't give up. If it was your parent, your brother, your spouse, your child—would you give up or keep looking?

"When you have a patient you have treated aggressively, to the best of your ability, and he or she is still not getting well, you have to ask, 'What else is going on?'"

Despite the logic of Horowitz's stand, it is still difficult for many to obtain a diagnosis of co-infection because—on the surface—there seems to be conflicting medical literature. But only on the surface. The confusion arises from the fact that many studies—like those at the CDC—restrict their criteria for Lyme disease for purposes of epidemiological tracking. They do *not* use the broader standards of medical diagnosis, and therefore fail to include some of the sickest patients. The key, says Horowitz, is for physicians—and medical consumers—to educate themselves regarding the possibility of emerging diseases and co-infections.

This type of relationship between doctor and patient creates an alliance that, at its best, can move mountains.

4.

Developing a Therapeutic Alliance

Kinship is healing; we are physicians to each other.

—Oliver Sacks, *Awakenings*

During the mid-1800s, the Countess Rosa Branka, of Poland, upon being diagnosed as having breast cancer, decided to take matters into her own hands—literally. Distrustful of the doctors, she amassed surgical instruments and performed surgery on herself, excising the cancerous lump. She lived another twenty-one years in good health.

While not many people would resort to the countess's drastic measures, the relationship between doctors and patients can be strained to the breaking point at a time when the two should work closely together. As one mother of a Lyme sufferer said: "The easy stuff they can treat. It's how they handle the difficult illnesses that lets you know the kind of doctor you have. This is when you get to see the heart and soul and guts of your doctor."

In approaching Lyme disease, as with any complicated illness, the doctor needs to throw away the "medical cookbook" and get to work as a detective, piecing together the clues to the final diagnosis. This may require an adjustment in practice and attitude, not only among the doctors involved but for the patients as well.

A major change over the last dozen years that affects the doctor-patient relationship is the accessibility and widespread use of the Internet. Many patients, fed up with intolerable waits, mini-appointments with rushed doctors, and the inability to reach a medical professional to ask questions, have turned to the Web for help. Instead of calling the office, patients are logging on. This is both good and bad.

There are a lot of excellent medical information sites on the Internet (see appendix C). There is also a lot of misinformation, because anyone with a point of view—whether supported by science or just a next-door neighbor's opinion—can have a website. And when we're talking about your health, wrong information can mean the difference between a cure and a chronic condition.

In speaking with both physicians and Lyme patients across the country, I have been able to categorize the ways in which a good working relationship can be sabotaged.

HOW PATIENTS OBSTRUCT
THE DOCTOR-PATIENT RELATIONSHIP

1. The "It's my doctor's job to keep me well" attitude.
This type of attitude leads patients to abdicate responsibility for good health practices. It allows them to smoke, drink to excess, and ignore good dietary recommendations, thereby sabotaging both antibiotic treatment and the immune system.

As medical consumers—and we must think of ourselves that way—it is *our* job to keep ourselves well; it is the doctor's job to find out what is wrong when we are unwell and make *recommendations* to "fix" us.

2. Diagnosing oneself and demanding specific therapy.
There have been a profusion of articles on Lyme disease as the problem has intensified in recent years. The media blitz, coupled with many physicians' confusion over diagnosis and treatment and the possible professional ramifications for them, has contributed to diagnostic decisions being made by informed patients even before speaking with a doctor. There is no doubt that many patients have been better informed than their doctors regarding

this disease. By the same token, the doctor must have a healthy skepticism and eliminate other possibilities as well. If you find a doctor who is informed on Lyme, let him do the job he was trained to do. Remember, other diseases must be ruled out.

3. Concealing important information.
There are patients who will say only what they think the doctor wants to hear, whether to save embarrassment, to cover up some "health sin," or simply to be liked. Some patients who have been doctoring themselves with homeopathic medicines and supplements, which can change body chemistry, will leave out this vital information. Some who have already diagnosed themselves will recite classic symptoms whether they have these symptoms or not, just to support their own diagnosis. This clouds the issue and further complicates the doctor's assessment. Real honesty is called for here—this is your life at stake.

4. Not providing enough information; being misleading.
A variation of the above, this is where a patient may evaluate the symptoms, prioritize them, and give the doctor only the top several, those bothering him the most. In some cases, particularly with Lyme, it may be the symptoms left out that clinch the diagnosis. This is a good example of where constructing a symptom log/journal will assist the doctor in accurately appraising the situation.

5. Talking too much about irrelevant issues.
One of the signs of disseminated Lyme is that patients tend to suffer from "motor mouth," chatting aimlessly but passionately about their symptoms, their relationships with others, and their treatment at the hands of others. While this can be a red flag for the examining physician, it can also misdirect the doctor's attention if it's done intentionally.

6. Belittling the entire medical profession.
One patient, upon meeting a new doctor, began his interview by telling the doctor what crooks most doctors were, how they

charged high prices just to pay for their cars and vacations, and ended with his favorite "joke": "You know what they call a guy who graduates at the bottom of his medical class, don't you? . . . Doctor!" Needless to say, the physician involved was not highly motivated to keep this man as a patient.

Doctors are only human (just ask their spouses!), and treating patients and curing illness is how they make a living. While some do take advantage, most are honestly interested in relieving suffering. They are entitled to charge for their services and will react in a human way when confronted by an obnoxious patient.

7. Patients who take advantage—or just plain take.
People who take objects from the doctor's office, ask to use the doctor's phone for an important call and then conduct business transactions or chat with relatives, or ask for use of the office equipment do nothing to strengthen the doctor-patient partnership.

HOW DOCTORS SABOTAGE
THE DOCTOR-PATIENT RELATIONSHIP

1. Doctors frequently don't schedule enough time for patients.
Those doctors who routinely see Lyme disease patients emphasize that the initial visit should take anywhere from one to one and one-half hours. Many doctors tend to overbook because of patient no-shows. Others have to work in emergencies. Still others find that patients have misled the booking receptionist regarding the extent of their symptoms and problems. Whatever the reason, it's normal for a sick patient to wait up to an hour to be seen. Then, when the patient finally is seen, the doctor is so frazzled that the patient is rushed through symptoms to "make up" for the tight schedule. This is not a new complaint, but it leads to the next problem.

2. Doctors don't listen.
Surprisingly, many doctors themselves will admit that as a whole, doctors don't listen well. As the patient starts talking, the

doctor is already mentally running through disease pathologies to quickly come up with the right answer. Doctors are also often guilty of taking outside calls during an examination, scheduling everything from restaurant reservations to auto repairs, and—*the* big problem regarding Lyme—many doctors deny there is even a possibility of Lyme disease and refuse to listen to what their patients have to say about it.

This denial on the part of ill-informed physicians has been responsible for the late diagnosis of Lyme, resulting in the permanent disability of thousands of men, women, and children.

During training, medical students are taught to ask the patient at some point, "What do *you* think the problem is?" Many times, the patient's observations can be helpful in finding the correct diagnosis.

3. Doctors show off to intimidate.
Before Dr. X sees a patient for the first time, the office receptionist hands the patient not only a "new patient information form" but a public relations release on the doctor as well. This lists his accomplishments, speeches, publications, and awards. "By the time the doctor walked in, I felt as though I should stand and applaud," said one, now former, patient, "let alone bother such an important person with my mundane aches and pains."

Although it is important to know that one's doctor is competent, more will be revealed by his willingness to listen to the patient and treat him respectfully than by using deliberately confusing language, medicalese, and press releases to stun the patient into subservience. An attitude of superiority is a large obstacle to the diagnosis of Lyme—a disease that even the most informed researchers admit is a confusing puzzle. Big egos get in the way of following the clues.

4. Doctors take inadequate medical histories.
"All medical textbooks are written from patient histories," said Debra, a Maryland physician who suffers from Lyme. "I had a medical professor who used to say that all the time, but the fact

is, most doctors rush through the history and miss a lot of information that could help them make a good diagnosis. Then the one who pays is the patient."

Since the diagnosis of Lyme is a *clinical one*—that is, one made by the doctor based upon a variety of symptoms rather than reliance on tests—the medical history is one of the *most important* diagnostic tools the doctor will have at his disposal. The specifics of what should be included will be discussed later in this chapter.

5. Doctors become defensive when confronted with puzzling symptoms.

Lyme disease is not a snap diagnosis. A doctor cannot take a throat culture, wait fifteen minutes, and pronounce Lyme. It is a painstaking process for both doctor and patient, and there are few patients who can realistically expect a snap answer. Doctors who become defensive when patients suggest Lyme disease reveal more about their own insecurities and inadequacies than anything else. If a doctor reacts in this manner, the whole relationship needs to be reevaluated.

6. Doctors don't believe the patient.

"I told him about the rash and the rest of the symptoms," said Clare. "He told me I must be reading too many newspaper articles."

"I gave my doctor my list of symptoms. She told me that I would be okay when my husband wasn't working the night shift anymore and we had a regular sex life again," said Dina.

"I told the doctor that I keep getting headaches that don't go away, that I had a stiff neck, pain in my knees, and was having trouble reading. And it all started after a field trip to a state park. He told me that being a kid was tough today and that I was just having growing pains," said Mark, a thirteen-year-old Lyme patient.

Unfortunately, these are not isolated incidents. Too many patients report that an early diagnosis (and therefore a cure) was hampered by doctors not believing what they were told. Patients' complaints were dismissed as everything from "growing pains" (kids), to "menopause" (even in women from the late twenties through forty), to stress. It is demeaning to not be believed. More important, if the patient does have Lyme, it is also dangerous.

Since the diagnosis for Lyme disease must be a clinical one, both doctors and patients need to polish off their interpersonal skills, throw out all these obstacles to a good working relationship, and strive to form a productive alliance to combat this or any other complicated and puzzling disease.

THE THERAPEUTIC ALLIANCE

Dr. Ken Liegner's office is right in the heart of one of the most beautiful areas of Westchester County, New York—and in one of the country's most hyperendemic areas for Lyme. A member of the medical advisory board for the Lyme Disease Association, he has been treating Lyme patients since 1985. He holds four medical patents, has testified before the New York State Assembly Committee on Health, and his more than three-dozen published research articles have earned him the respect of both academics and clinicians. His emphasis that Lyme is a clinical diagnosis includes detailed instructions for what he considers the most important diagnostic tool: the patient history, given in the context of a new alliance.

"The therapeutic alliance isn't really a new idea; it stems from psychoanalytic writings stretching way back," he says. "And it should not be unique to Lyme disease. You must have a therapeutic alliance to be successful. A doctor by him- or herself can't do anything; a doctor and patient cooperating can accomplish a lot."

Foremost in developing the alliance on the doctor's side is allowing adequate time for the initial visit and the detailed patient history that must be taken, particularly if there is any question or suspicion of Lyme disease. "Some patients have very long, puzzling histories with symptoms that go over many years and may seem odd. We have to take the time to listen. There is also an art to eliciting a history.

"We are taught in med school to listen to a patient, but a lot of us forget it along the way. We really have to listen carefully to what the patient is saying, not show how smart we are by cutting off their sentences and finishing it. We need to process that information and then ask pointed questions to elicit the kind of information that the patient may not have even realized is important."

This information includes an expanded geographic history of the patient's vocations, vacations, camping and sporting activities, and even daily activities.

One little girl who contracted Lyme was getting progressively sicker. She remained undiagnosed because the physician in charge just couldn't see how, living in a semiurban environment, the child could have been exposed. It wasn't until another physician had her recount a typical day that it was revealed that, in order to catch her school bus, she took a shortcut through two hundred yards of underbrush, stacked wood, and mouse-infested shacks. A subsequent tick collection in that area revealed a high infection rate.

"In order to ask the right questions, a doctor has to have a good understanding of the disease. Because Lyme is so complicated and can present in so many different ways, a doctor has to have a good grasp of the wide range of symptoms that Lyme can produce. The simple, classic symptoms can be recognized by anyone who has bothered to read anything at all on Lyme, but there are so many odd, bizarre, and one-of-a-kind symptoms, a doctor has to at least be aware of the possibilities that exist.

"For this reason, you need a good grasp of medical knowledge generally so you don't go barking up the wrong tree. Just as bad as diagnosing Lyme that isn't there, is failing to diagnose a case that is."

Liegner admits that many doctors shy away from dealing

with Lyme patients because it is at times a difficult, time-consuming relationship. Patients can be highly emotional and many are frustrated, having been bounced from specialist to specialist with decreasing empathy for the pain they are experiencing. Add in other resulting life stresses—financial, familial, and career-related—and you have some panicked and sick people transferring a lot of concerns onto the doctor's shoulders.

Liegner, a veteran researcher in the diagnosing and treatment of Lyme, utilizing both classic medical as well as adjunctive therapies when necessary, sometimes resorts to what he calls "the total push." This is when, he says, "you're confronted with a very sick person—you use every treatment modality available that is likely to help. This term has been used by psychoanalysts for years. It means, you don't stop, you don't give up, you try everything within your power to get that person well." And that type of dedication of purpose translates into confidence for the patient that his or her doctor is firmly in their corner.

Liegner emphasizes that doctors need to return to trusting their own powers of observation—something that makes many of them, who would rather rely on the empirical results of a test, feel uncomfortable. "And a delay in diagnosis can result in long-term, chronic infection," he said. "People need to be made aware of this—both doctors and the general public. Yes, doctors need to be skeptical, especially if they are presented with a patient who has self-diagnosed, but to deny the possibility of Lyme entirely is dangerous and potentially injurious."

The medical history, the physical examination, and the relevant tests are all needed to contribute to a diagnosis of Lyme. The most controversial of the three, however, is the testing procedure and its erratic, and too frequently unreliable results. In researching Lyme, great emphasis is being placed on discovering reliable tests.

5.

Translating Those Tests into English

The diagnostic problems surrounding Lyme disease are derived primarily from the fact that there have been no tests that could simply and positively detect the *Borrelia burgdorferi* spirochete, thus confirming Lyme and initiating the traditional therapeutic process.

From Tufts University in Massachusetts to Stony Brook in New York to Tulane University to the NIH-sponsored mecca of scientific research—Rocky Mountain Labs in Hamilton, Montana—specialists from a dozen different fields are pooling their knowledge to pick apart the infectious spirochete, infamous for its ability to transform its appearance chemically, in much the same way a criminal might change clothes and hair color to evade detection and capture.

For this reason, the primary tests for Lyme have measured the body's response to the foreign particles—a measurement of antibodies—rather than picking up the organism itself.

In scientific labs across the country, it has been said that the ideal or "gold standard" test would be to simply be able to culture and grow the *Borrelia burgdorferi* spirochete outside the human body as proof of its presence *in* the body. We will discuss a little later how such tests have recently been developed and may be available for future use. But, although many bacteria may be able to reproduce every twenty minutes, *B. burgdorferi* has been found to regenerate in a range spanning twelve hours to eighteen days, similar to the rate of the organism that causes TB. In reviewing the damage it inflicts, one can assess just how

potent small amounts of this spirochete can be, as well as how
difficult it might be to find.

Anyone experiencing a difficult-to-diagnose illness becomes con-
versant in the medical jargon of diagnostic tests, blood counts,
and assays (the chemical analyses of substances). Entering the
world of Lyme disease is no different. Ranging from the simplest
and most commonly used tests to the more complex and more
accurate assays currently going through confirmation trials, the
tests listed below may assist in determining infection.

THE BASIC TESTS

When infection is present in the human body, the immune system produces complex substances called antibodies to neutralize
or destroy the invading organisms (the antigen). Each type of
antibody, however, recognizes only the type of antigen that pro-
vokes its formation. In theory, then, if one were to measure the
body's production of Lyme antibodies, it would seem reasonable
to assume that Lyme was indeed present.

   Three problems arise regarding such a test for Lyme disease,
however. The first is that even if you watched a tick that you knew
to be infected with *Borrelia burgdorferi* feed on your body for
twenty-four hours and then took a blood test, the test would come
out negative. This is because it takes the body from three to six
weeks or longer to begin to produce the antibodies to fight the
infection. During that time, a person can begin to exhibit definite
Lyme symptoms, yet will test negative for the disease—despite
the fact of sure infection. This would result in a false negative test.

   The second problem is that the Lyme spirochete is made up
of thousands of foreign proteins, some of which are similar to
the proteins of other bacteria. It is possible that a person with
another type of bacterial infection—and who has antibodies to
that infection or co-infection—would test positive for Lyme

even if he or she did not have it. This is called cross-reactivity and could result in a false positive test.

Finally, some researchers believe that, particularly in cases where a person was infected months or years prior to the testing, the body's immune system may be so beaten down that only the most highly specialized and sensitive test could detect the antibodies left after the infection has destroyed the original chemical "soldiers."

Further complications arise if the patient has recently taken antibiotics, steroids, or anti-inflammatory drugs like prednisone, which could inhibit the production of antibodies. New research has shown that the spirochete has the ability to hide within the host body's cell walls, adopt a cyst form, or change its protein makeup so as to be unrecognizable to the appropriate antibodies. In addition, the reliability of test results is also only as good as the labs and technicians doing the work—various working conditions and mass-produced test kits operate on the sensitivity of the chemicals involved and often produce varied results. More than a few doctors have complained that they have sent portions of the same blood sample to two different labs only to get two different results, and a recent survey showed that approximately half of the labs cannot reproduce their own original results from the same samples.

It is obvious, then, why many doctors will either attempt to diagnose Lyme without bothering with antibody tests or will run tests but give little credence to the results.

The most commonly administered tests, if your doctor suspects Lyme could be present, are the IFA, the ELISA, the Western Blot, or the PCR.

IFA   Stands for immunofluorescent assay. This test can be performed with equipment already in place in most laboratories. It specifically measures total immunoglobulin (Ig), IgM, and IgG (different proteins) antibodies. During various stages of Lyme, the antibody levels will rise. If a patient is presenting arthritic or neurologic symptoms, for example, the IgG or IgM antibody levels could be elevated.

ELISA   This enzyme-linked immunosorbent assay has been easier to standardize than the IFA, is usually considered the first test to administer for suspected Lyme, and is part of the CDC's two-test protocol. However, the group responsible for proficiency testing for the College of American Pathologists (CAP) recently came to the conclusion that the currently available ELISA assays for Lyme disease do not have adequate sensitivity to meet the requirements of the CDC because they were not designed by the manufacturers to be sensitive at the 95 percent level required for screening.

ELISA tests for IgG and IgM antibodies, indicating their presence through a color change, but these results are notorious for varying from lab to lab. Much work needs to be done to standardize the basic ELISA's precision for Lyme antibody detection. Some doctors and labs are now employing a new and exciting variation of the ELISA called a C6 Peptide ELISA (sometimes referred to as the VlsE C6 ELISA), which is not only demonstrating increased sensitivity to all strains and species of the Lyme disease spirochete both here and in Europe but is Lyme-specific.

Developed by Dr. Mario Philipp and his group at the Tulane National Primate Research Center in Covington, Louisiana, the test, which is manufactured by Immunetics in Cambridge, Massachusetts, and is available through most diagnostic labs, has won approval from the U.S. Food and Drug Administration (FDA). A C6-based ELISA has been recently evaluated by the CDC and judged as good in sensitivity and specificity as the two-tiered test approach the CDC recommends. Dr. Philipp, who has dedicated the last five years to researching and developing a gold-standard diagnostic test for Lyme at his laboratory deep in bayou country, across the vast Lake Ponchartrain, is cautiously optimistic about the C6 test's future: "The C6 peptide is part of a lipoprotein, VlsE, which sits on the surface membrane of the spirochete. Parts of this protein are changed by the spirochete as it infects the host, but other portions, C6 included, stay constant and stimulate an early and strong antibody response. This is why the C6 test is so sensitive, as it detects antibody very early in the infection. It is also very specific for Lyme."

Philipp says that aside from it being successful so far in reacting specifically to a wide variety of spirochetal strains, another advantage to the C6 ELISA is that it is comparatively easy for a laboratory to make. It also can be used with patients who still have antibodies to the Lyme vaccine, as it does not cross-react with these antibodies. The C6 ELISA will not detect co-infections, such as babesiosis, but it may prove to have a valuable role in detecting and diagnosing Lyme disease.

Western Blot This test is often used to confirm borderline-positive serology or in evaluating false positives. It is the most useful test in revealing Lyme disease. It separates the proteins by molecular weight, illustrating them in chartlike bands, some of which are specific for *Borrelia burgdorferi.*

The key to the successful use of the Western Blot is that it must be performed in a quality laboratory that charts and reports all of the bands, not just the present "CDC-specific" bands. What you should know is that the criteria developed by the CDC concerning the Western Blot are stringent, relying on only up to three bands on the IgM blot and up to ten bands on the IgG blot out of the ninety-nine available. If fewer than five bands are positive, the lab may report the test as negative. But the CDC—and I can't stress this strongly enough throughout the book—sets criteria strictly for limited epidemiological tracking purposes, not for clinical diagnostics. This limitation ignores the diversity of individual immune responses.

You should not only insist upon a Western Blot if Lyme disease is suspected but also make sure that the lab your doctor sends it to is one that develops and reports *all* the bands present, not just the CDC-specific bands on both the IgM and IgG. Two labs that are meticulous about their testing protocols are Medical Diagnostic Laboratories in Mt. Laurel, New Jersey, and

IGeneX in Palo Alto, California. The lab at the State University of New York at Stony Brook will report all bands present on the blot if this is requested at the time of submission of the specimen.

The Lumbar Puncture   Also called a spinal tap, a lumbar puncture drains a small sample of cerebral spinal fluid from the lower spine. A needle is inserted between the vertebrae (backbone) in the lower back and into the space containing the spinal fluid. This is a test that frightens many people who have heard horror stories, but it is rare that something goes wrong. This test is important for the following reasons: the physician may be able to garner some additional information that will help make the diagnosis by either detecting DNA from a spirochete directly or culturing a spirochete from the fluid; it is an important tool for ruling out other diseases; it can detect co-infections which also need to be treated; and it can reveal any abnormalities in the cerebral spinal fluid.

The Lyme Urine Antigen-Capture Test   Detects small blister-like cells (called blebs) given off from the outer membrane of the infectious spirochete. These blebs become free-floating agents and are present in the urine of a patient infected with Lyme. The assay itself is a two-step procedure employing two different immune system proteins that search out and bind to proteins of the infectious organisms in a manner analogous to a lock and key. The presence of these Lyme proteins is a definite indication of infection. Two versions of this test have been on the market, but these may not be available for clinical use at the present time, though this could change.

The Fluorescent In-Situ Hybridization (FISH) Assay   This relatively new test was developed at and is available exclusively through IgeneX, a specialty immunology laboratory and research facility in Palo Alto, California. Headed by Dr. Nick Harris, a board-certified immunologist, IgeneX's FISH assay is an RNA-based test that is able to detect *Babesia* parasites in those who might also be infected with Lyme. It has been approved for use throughout the country.

Borreliacidal Antibody Assay (Gunderson Test)   Developed by University of Wisconsin Medical School professor Ronald Schell, Ph.D., and Gunderson Lutheran Medical research scientist Steve Callister at the Gundersen Clinic in La Crosse, Wisconsin. It is a promising test that detects bacteria-killing antibodies found in the blood of Lyme patients. So far, there does not appear to be cross-reactivity and the results suggested that the borreliacidal assay might differentiate active infection from past exposure. This would represent a major scientific breakthrough in that it would eliminate the need for the present CDC two-tiered system of testing and serve as the elusive "gold-standard" that would address why certain patients, even after treatment, are still ill. Despite performing well in CDC trials, the test is still not readily available in most parts of the country.

The Quantitative Rapid Identification of *Borrelia burgdorferi* (Q-RIBb)   Developed by Dr. Jo Anne Whitaker, president and director of research for the Bowen Research and Training Institute in Palm Harbor, Florida, and validated and refined independently by Dr. Lida Mattman, professor emeritus of biology at Wayne State University in Detroit, and Dr. Steven Phillips of Connecticut, this is another promising new test, presently experimental, designed to culture Lyme disease spirochetes from the blood rather than look for antibodies. Dr. Whitaker says the test is in the final stages of being patented, but in the meantime is helping isolate *Borrelia* in the blood and cerebral spinal fluid for those doctors and patients who request it. She also takes digital photos to document the findings and provides a quantitative analysis of the organisms. The test can be concentrated to pinpoint babesiosis and ehrlichiosis as well.

The Multiplex PCR Assay   IGeneX has developed a three-step, nucleic acid-based PCR diagnostic assay that is proving to be even more sensitive than the standard in clinical trials and has increased specificity even when the patient has previously been on an antibiotic regimen.

Finally, it is important to undergo formal detailed psychological testing, particularly if you are experiencing any neurological problems. Psychological testing by a knowledgeable psychiatrist provides important objective data and patterns that can be compared over time to determine the efficacy of the treatment your doctor prescribes.

DETECTION THROUGH DNA

One of the more sensitive tests to be developed is the polymerase chain reaction (PCR), which seeks to identify portions of the DNA (the nucleic acid forming the main component of living cells) from the spirochete itself by using urine, blood, or cerebral spinal fluid samples from the infected patient. Detection of the spirochete's DNA would definitely confirm that a patient has Lyme. The one drawback to PCR, thus far, is that the test itself is so slow (results can take a week) and sensitive that a change of temperature in the lab, the proximity of one specimen to another, and even the level of dust and the technician's handling of the samples can influence the outcome.

Dr. Manfred Bayer is a tall, distinguished-looking scientist who spends his days as director of the Lyme Disease Laboratory of the Fox Chase Institute for Cancer Research in Philadelphia, working through the problems of PCR sensitivity. Bayer, a neurologist from Hamburg, Germany, specializing in tropical medicine and virology, is internationally known for his work on bacterial cell surface receptors. Bayer's courtliness doesn't mask the intensity with which he attacks the Lyme disease detection problem. Bayer describes his research:

"There are certain areas of the DNA strand that are very specific to the microorganism from which it comes; other areas are not so specific," says Bayer. "We are only interested in the *Borrelia burgdorferi* specific sequences. What one makes is an artificial DNA potion [or probe] that will recognize the specific DNA sequences to that organism [*B. burgdorferi*] taken from the test urine. Normally DNA is double stranded. We need to force it into a single strand [done through a heating process] and at that moment, the complementary artificial piece can find the complementary segment of the bacterial strand."

A continuation of the process involves the adding of an enzyme and several steps of heating and cooling in a reaction chamber; the result is the thousand- to millionfold reproduction of the DNA, which, if from infected fluid, can show spirochetal presence. PCR has allowed scientists to determine that specific portions of the spirochete DNA may affect different portions of the human body.

"The sensitivity of the PCR test is such that all it takes for results to be in question is one unwashed hand grabbing a tube contaminated from an outside source. Sometimes there are lots of these microorganisms out there that can contaminate the sample."

It is important, therefore, that any physician requesting a PCR to validate Lyme or any other illness be convinced that the laboratory handling such testing has protocols in place to guard against the variables that could render the test useless. The College of American Pathologists (CAP) proficiency program evaluates commercial labs that offer Lyme PCR testing. If the lab satisfies the CAP program, you can be reasonably assured that the results are valid and meaningful.

ROCKY MOUNTAIN LABORATORIES

Dwarfed by the majestic Bitterroot Mountains, the red-bricked, multibuilding complex that comprises Rocky Mountain Laboratories (RML) sits at the end of residential street in Hamilton, Montana, surrounded by a high chain-link fence topped with barbed wire. It is here that some of the world's most puzzling and debilitating diseases—mad cow disease, plague, hepatitis, AIDS, tuberculosis, and chlamydia—are studied, and cures are designed.

Here is where the ticks, obtained from the canyon visible in the distance, were ground up to make vaccines for Rocky Mountain spotted fever. And here is where a team of sixteen scientists labored full-time every day to understand the physiology of an organism so robust and virulent that its discoverer, Dr. Willy Burgdorfer, wryly commented, "It's a helluva bug and I'm sorry my name's on it."

It was at Rocky Mountain Labs, one of the National Institute of Allergy and Infectious Diseases' (NIAID) premiere satellite facilities, that Lyme disease served as a major focus of attention over the last decade. Thanks to the efforts of Drs. David Dorward, Claude Garon, Patti Rosa, William Whitmore, Richard Marconi, and Tom Schwann, among others, such tests as the Rocky Mountain Antigen Capture Assay and recombinant DNA tests were developed and helped in the diagnosing and treating of thousands of Lyme patients.

Rocky Mountain Labs' newest distinction is that, by the end of 2004, it will be one of only four scientific labs in the country equipped to handle the highest level of containment for deadly microbes, thanks to a $66 million federal allocation for bioterrorism research. While Lyme disease is still on the agenda, senior investigator Schwann says that the hot disease under the microscope now is relapsing fever, another tick-borne pathogen that is causing epidemics in many parts of the world, including the United States (see chapter 3).

NEUROLOGIC LYME DISEASE

While the ELISA and Western Blot are generally used to confirm a diagnosis of neurological involvement in Lyme disease, your physician may recommend several other tests to evaluate for neurological involvement.

Magnetic Resonance Imaging (MRI) Uses a magnetic field, radio waves, and a computer to create detailed image slices (cross sections) of the area. MRI technology produces better soft-tissue images than X ray and allows the physician to evaluate different types of tissue, as well as distinguish normal, healthy tissue from diseased tissue. It can not only detect tumors (for a differential diagnosis) but show damaged tissues. In neurologic Lyme disease, approximately 15 to 45 percent of patients' brains show spots of white matter, sometimes called UBOs or "unidentified bright objects," that can hamper normal brain function. These sometimes diminish with antibiotic treatment.

Single Photon Emission Computerized Tomography (SPECT) Like the MRI, this is an imaging device. The role of this procedure is to assess distribution of a radioactive isotope thought to relate to brain blood flow. It can help in evaluating memory loss, degenerative disease, strokes, and seizures. Brain SPECT scans may also be used to evaluate brain injury.

During the exam, the patient receives an intravenous injection of a tracer dose of radioactive material. The level of radioactivity is extremely low and has no side effects. The patient is required to lie flat on the back without moving for approximately thirty minutes to an hour. Using a special nuclear medicine camera, pictures of the brain are taken so the progress and distribution of the radioactive material in the brain can be recorded.

Positron Emission Tomography (PET) Another imaging tool and similar in procedure to the SPECT scan, PET can demonstrate biochemical or physiological processes involved in the brain's metabolism and function. This scan is at a higher resolution and provides a more detailed picture of the brain's abnormalities, including lesions resulting from *Borrelia* infection that has leached into the cerebral spinal fluid.

TESTS FOR DIFFERENTIAL DIAGNOSES

Since your doctor will be attempting to rule out other illnesses in the search for a diagnosis involving Lyme, several other tests are commonly ordered.

Lumbar Puncture   Doctors are divided over its efficacy for Lyme, since a negative result does not mean that Lyme isn't present. It is helpful, however, if the infection is being caused by some other infectious agent. The lumbar puncture *is not* done to rule in Lyme, it is done to rule out other diseases.

CAT scan   *CAT* is an abbreviation for computerized axial tomography. This is a painless diagnostic procedure in which hundreds of X rays of a specific area of the body are taken, then fed into a computer, which integrates them to present a very detailed view.

EEG   This is the electroencephalogram, which, through the measurement of electrical impulses in the brain, rules out abnormal brain activity leading to seizure disorders.

VERS   The VERS, or visual evoked responses, is a more sensitive test for MS.

Blood tests:

   Thyroid profile—to rule out thyroid disease

   ANA—used in collagen diseases, especially lupus

   VDRL-RPR—to rule out syphilis

   CBC—checks for anemia

   B_{12}-folate levels—low levels lead to mental confusion and neurologic defects

   In undiagnosed chronic Lyme, an immune system evaluation called T & B Cell Subsets will help explain symptoms caused by an immune system run amok.

The results from any of these tests aside, one aspect of Lyme is finally being recognized as an integral component of this disease. It is one of the most challenging to measure because its scope encompasses both the physical and the psychological, also one of the most difficult to accept and the most complicated to treat. This is the neuropsychiatric aspect of Lyme disease.

6.

"I'm Not Crazy, I Have Lyme!"

Living in a rural area of Pennsylvania, Lanie loved to spend the time when she wasn't working at the Sylvania plant tending her garden. She thinks that might have been what did her in. First she got severe pain in her joints and pain in her back, then a stiff neck and terrible headaches. Her doctor told the fifty-two-year-old that she had fibrositis, brought on by passing out at the plant and banging her head.

Whatever the cause, Lanie's energy level had been sapped, her production level at work was detrimentally low, and she was experiencing sleep disturbances. She became terribly depressed and cried easily. Her doctor put her on prednisone, muscle relaxers, and sleeping pills, but her body continued to fall apart. Pressing for a reevaluation, she was told she had fibromyalgia and depression and that she'd have to live with them.

"My husband, who was having similar symptoms, was going to retire to take care of me," she said. "I kept having more symptoms and thought I was going to lose my mind. I had stomach pain, my arms were getting weak. The doctor didn't believe me. I had a wonderful life and it was falling apart." Then she saw an article in *Outdoor Life* magazine on Lyme disease and her symptoms began to fall into place. She sought out a Lyme support group, even though it met more than a hundred miles from her home, and listened to an epidemiologist give a presentation that opened her eyes further. Most of those Lyme patients had to travel out of state for knowledgeable treatment. She went to see her local doctor again and he gave her ulcer medication. "I asked for a Lyme test and he told me he didn't want to even discuss it. He said I was being ridiculous."

Lanie returned home, feeling demoralized. She took the medicine for her stomach and reacted with Bell's palsy. She called another doctor, who recommended a spinal tap. When she asked if she could have a Lyme test, he said, "If you think you know more than I do, go find yourself another doctor."

"Then I had no doctor, and no one who could tell me about Lyme. I was so nervous by that time, I was dealing with such pain and pressure in my head, that I just snapped one afternoon. I started to cry hysterically on the back porch—everything just seemed to come crashing down on me and I had to let it out. Well, the neighbors heard me wailing and called the police. When the police came, they pushed me down on the ground and put me in a straitjacket. I kept yelling at them, 'I'm not crazy! I have Lyme disease, I have Lyme disease!' but they wouldn't listen. They drove me to the county hospital and put me on the psycho ward.

"They got ahold of my husband, but it didn't do any good. I had to stay there for five days, by law, before they could let me out. They wanted to do an evaluation. They gave me Compazine and Elavil, and I had an allergic reaction to the Compazine—my tongue swelled and I could hardly breathe. The psychiatrist came in and scolded me that if I didn't stop complaining, he was going to confine me to the state mental hospital.

"While I was there, a medical student who was working there came to see me. He said he had the same kind of symptoms I had and we compared notes. Finally, on the fifth day, my husband came with a lawyer who confronted the doctors with all kinds of supportive information on Lyme and they let me out.

"I finally got to a doctor—had to go to Indiana—and began treatment. You really are treated as if you are crazy, and you begin to doubt your own sanity. Some days it was really hard to hang on."

■ ■ ■

Not all tales are as dramatic as Lanie's, but talk to a thousand Lyme patients and you will get a thousand variations of the same story: people who are normally easygoing become moody and belligerent; those who are outgoing become lethargic; mood swings cause the breakup of marriages and career relationships; the inability to concentrate results in job losses, plunging grades in school, and accidents; short-term memory loss affects habits and speech; and everywhere there is depression, a loss of self-esteem, and suicidal thoughts from people who have never had a history of such things.

Like that other infamous spirochetal illness, syphilis, Lyme disease has a definitive array of psychological symptoms as well as physical ones. Depending upon the lag time between the tick bite and treatment, these symptoms can be either mild or severe.

Although the CDC and most doctors and researchers now concede that the *Borrelia* spirochete can invade every system of the body, including the cerebral spinal fluid that flows to the brain, not enough attention has been paid to the neuropsychiatric aspects of Lyme disease. It is often these symptoms that present the greatest impediment to a person living his or her life and coping with other aspects of the illness. After all, if your knee or stomach hurts but you can think clearly, you could still educate yourself, ask questions, communicate with others, and even hope to carry out daily responsibilities in whatever capacity your body allows.

But with neurologic Lyme—and the longer one has Lyme the more likely it is that the spirochetes will invade the brain—a person becomes incapacitated in a more fundamental way. Whether adult or child, he or she cannot think clearly, may suffer seizures, cannot remember the simplest things, may display obsessive-compulsive disorder, may be overwhelmed with a hypersensitivity to sound and light, can get lost in familiar places, cannot concentrate, may exhibit mood swings, sleep disturbances, and irritability, and finally can deteriorate into anxiety and depression. A recent study, published in the *Journal of Neuropsychiatry and Clinical Neurosciences* on children with chronic Lyme, revealed that 41 percent had suicidal thoughts and 11 percent had made a suicidal gesture. The percentages of adults experiencing suicidal feelings may be higher and adults may be more likely to carry out a successful suicide attempt.

The symptoms, coupled with all the other reasons for misdiagnosis and late diagnosis, often prompt doctors to tell Lyme patients, "Look, there's nothing wrong with you physically—it's all in your head. Go see a psychiatrist." This scenario has been replayed with such frequency that it has become a standing joke among Lyme patients: They say that if your doctor finally tells you to go see a shrink, that's the confirmation that you have Lyme disease! And as one psychiatrist wryly commented, "We are at the end of a long line of doctors. When nobody else can figure out what's wrong with a patient, they send him to us."

Far from being humorous, however, the mind-body connection is one of the more difficult aspects with which to deal, both when seeking a proper diagnosis and when just attempting to cope on a daily basis. The Lyme infection apparently wreaks havoc with those neurons affecting the personality and emotional balance.

But when does the cucumber evolve into the pickle? In other words, when does the physiological effect of neurologic Lyme become an organic psychiatric problem and the emotional impact of the physical illness have a reactive psychological consequence?

Contrary to a prevailing belief, those who are felled by Lyme are not hypochondriacs looking for attention. In fact, there is a lot of denial that goes on—first over physical symptoms, then when the possibility of Lyme disease arises, and finally when psychological symptoms appear. This is not only a threatening aspect of the illness itself, but if the patient has had to fight for a diagnosis and treatment, the vicious cycle of doubt, self-doubt, and alienation and depression figures largely into the struggle for regaining health.

This is difficult enough for an adult who has a track record of wellness and a strong identity to fall back on, but when Lyme attacks children and teens the psychological presentations are intermingled with a number of other developmental issues. So though all of the following symptoms apply to young people as well, I will deal with the specific psychological effects and symptoms of Lyme on children and teens in chapters 8 and 9.

ZEROING IN ON THE PSYCHOLOGICAL ASPECTS

"When I asked for a Lyme test, the doctor asked me if I was afraid that my husband was going to leave me," said thirty-two-year-old Linda, who had been suffering from fatigue, joint pain, headaches, and swollen glands. "She said my symptoms were psychosomatic and would go away when our sex life picked up.

"I remember being on a school trip with my daughter on the bus and suddenly I felt as though I was in a fog and everyone else was far away. I could hear the noise and it was irritating, but I couldn't connect. I thought, 'My God, I *am* going crazy.' When a doctor tells you, 'It's all in your head,' you try to justify all your symptoms.

"It took two years and five doctors to figure out I had Lyme disease. It put a strain on my marriage, on my family relationships, and there were times that I was so depressed that I wondered if I'd finish out my days in the cuckoo ward. I've lost friends, self-esteem, and two years of my life, and I'm just hoping that someday soon I'll get back to normal. I ran into that first doctor recently. When I told her that I was being successfully treated for Lyme, she told me that I was crazy. That I didn't have Lyme disease and never did."

Fortunately for neurologic Lyme patients like Linda, doctors are beginning to realize that Lyme disease does cause certain psychological changes with which one must be prepared to deal. A good portion of the credit for bringing this to the attention of the medical community goes to Dr. Brian Fallon, an NIH fellow and associate professor of clinical psychiatry with the New York

State Psychiatric Institute at Columbia University in New York City, who has won international recognition for making the psychiatric aspects of Lyme disease a passionate area of study. As well as being author of cutting-edge studies on the neuropsychiatric aspects of Lyme, Dr. Fallon has been appointed head of the first national Lyme Disease Research Center at Columbia University and funded in large part by Time For Lyme of Greenwich, Connecticut (see chapter 21), and the Lyme Disease Association.

Fallon's passion for the suffering of Lyme patients began with a flood of referrals from doctors who couldn't figure out what was wrong with their patients and thus concluded "it must be in their heads." He has now presented papers at medical conferences both in the United States and in Europe, and has, together with Drs. Burrascano, Liegner, and Jennifer Nields, initiated surveys and studies that are serving as the yardstick for evaluating Lyme patients psychologically.

Based on treatment experience and the results of the nationally distributed survey, the neuropsychiatric symptoms of Lyme include:

- Major depression
- Extreme fatigue
- Emotional instability (crying easily)
- Increased irritability and mood swings
- Sensitivity to light
- Sleep disturbances (insomnia; too much sleep)
- Memory problems
- Getting lost in familiar places
- Dyslexia-type reversals
- Significant loss of libido
- Night terrors
- Panic attacks
- Ferocious nightmares
- Suicidal thoughts
- Mental fog
- Disorientation

- Feelings of rage
- Violent thoughts
- Abnormalities of taste
- Abnormalities of smell
- Heightened sensitivity to vibrations and noise
- Depersonalization
- Spatial problems
- Appetite changes (bulimia, anorexia)
- Obsessive-compulsive acts
- Seizures
- Lack of concentration
- Bell's palsy

Secondary psychological problems arising from Lyme include feelings of inadequacy, low self-esteem, bitterness, guilt, and alienation, as well as doubting one's sanity ("I feel as though I'm losing my mind" is a commonly heard phrase).

"The experience of Lyme is such that a patient will have unusual symptoms to the point of being disbelieved by doctors and family and finally disbelieving him- or herself," said Fallon. "This disease follows a waxing and waning course. You can't predict how you're going to feel the next day, next month, or next year. Family, friends, and schools say, 'Why are you okay one day and not the next?' Add to this that many patients have negative blood tests so there may be uncertainty of a Lyme diagnosis, and then you also have fear—fear of losing one's job, fear of losing health, and fear of losing the support of family and friends who may be supportive during the first month of the illness, but when this goes on and on, friends and family may get pretty tired of it.

"Lyme patients also feel a loss of control, not only of their bodies and feelings, but also the ability to anticipate and predict the future. Then they deal with shame, guilt, and finally anger directed at doctors and family members.

"Often psychiatrists are being asked to see these patients before a diagnosis of Lyme disease is made," said Fallon. "Incorrectly labeling these patients as having functional depression or hypochondriasis or a somatization disorder may result in delayed antibiotic treatment. Such a delay can lead to further dissemination of infection, severe disability, and possible chronic neurological damage.

"Because of the rapid increase of Lyme disease in the country (more than 40 percent in the last two years, according to the CDC's admittedly conservative numbers), it's important for mental health professionals as well as other health professionals to be aware of these psychological manifestations. Oftentimes, if you don't have the advantage of the tick bite and rash, these patients aren't picked up as having Lyme disease until too late."

Although the psychological manifestations of the disease are dismissed by some as "Lyme anxiety," that term cannot begin to cover the varied and intense personality changes that accompany Lyme, particularly in people who have no history of those types of changes. *The most common presentation is a feeling of depression.* And although some may simply experience uncomfortable feelings of doom, others experience a more sustained version, even to the point of gross debilitation.

LYME AND DEPRESSION

In an article for *Emergency Medicine,* Dr. Edwin H. Cassem, chief of psychiatry at Massachusetts General Hospital in Boston and professor of psychiatry at Harvard Medical School, wrote that classic depression has eight specific criteria, which he reduced to a mnemonic: Sig E. Caps (a doctor's prescription for energy capsules). This stands for *sleep, interest, guilt, energy, concentration, appetite, psychomotor,* and *suicidal ideas.* If a patient displays symptoms in four of the eight areas, he or she meets the criteria for major depression.

According to Fallon's study, which was done only on seropositive patients, 85 percent experienced sleep disturbances; 94 percent experienced extreme fatigue; 84 percent suffered from irritability and agitation; 24 percent had worked through suicidal plans, while many more admitted to suicidal thoughts; and 83 percent had difficulty with concentration and memory. Although specific questions regarding interests were not posed, most patients reported a significant loss of libido and interest in other aspects of their lives. Most also commented on the guilt they felt for the length of time they were ill; for the physical, emotional, and financial toll their illness was taking on their families; and for not being able to "will" themselves well. And just as with the physical presentations of Lyme, the psychological disturbances affect a patient's whole family.

Tom found his diagnosis on a milk carton. The thirty-eight-year-old was a self-employed furniture maker who loved to camp and study ecology with an artisan's eye. It could have been during one of his forays into the countryside or even while coaching his Little League team that Tom was bitten by the tick. As both his body and personality deteriorated (he was so dizzy, he felt "high" all the time), he made the rounds of doctors who threw tranquilizers at him to help him cope with "stress." By this time, the pressure in his head was so bad that he would curl up on the floor in a fetal position and cry. He couldn't bear noise and would lash out at those closest to him for the simplest comments or questions.

When he saw Lyme disease information on a milk carton one morning, a light went on. Tom finally found a knowledgeable doctor and began treatment, but ask any member of his family what it is like to have someone with Lyme in the house and there is a tussle over who'll answer first. "I hate it," the thirteen-year-old says angrily. "It's the pits," admits Tom's wife. "I don't even want to think about it," agrees the nine-year-old.

"This kind of thing, it affects families for life," says Tom's wife, Di. "The kids never know what kind of mood he's going to be in, so everyone walks on eggshells. The youngest one now hits himself in the head when he gets frustrated because he saw his father do that so often. I got to the point that I was crying all the time.

"One of the hardest things to deal with is that he doesn't *look* sick. Sick people are supposed to look sick, and everyone has sympathy for them. With Lyme, you can look pretty normal even though your body and mind seem to be falling apart on the inside, and people think you're a hypochondriac, making up symptoms."

Not being believed because one doesn't "look sick" adds to the Lyme patient's frustrations and self-doubts, but the lack of control over one's body—and mind—adds to overall depression.

Scott also does not look sick. In fact, if one were to look around a room full of people, this muscular man with blond hair, clear skin, and an engaging smile would be last on your list of sickly types. But for the last two years he has waged a battle with Lyme that has taken a toll both physically and emotionally.

"I was driving down a street in my neighborhood, where I've lived all my life," said the twenty-seven-year-old, who owns and operates his own landscaping business. "And suddenly, I was lost! I didn't recognize a thing. That is so scary! I mean, I lived on that street for years, and in an instant, I couldn't figure out where I was. I know of another guy with Lyme who put his hand on the doorknob and suddenly he couldn't remember how to turn the key to open the door. When these kinds of things happen, you really have to fight to remain stable. You go from being an active, competent person to being afraid to go out and even be with people because you don't know if you're going to forget words when you open your mouth."

This uncertainty and lack of control have forced many adult Lyme patients back into a dependent position, whether living at their parents' home again or simply having to depend on others in the household to do the simplest personal tasks. This contributes to feelings of guilt, worthlessness, and resentment, which can spill over onto the very people who are helping. Adding to the difficulty with relationships is the loss of libido that many people experience.

LOSS OF LIBIDO

"I feel as though I've been castrated," said Kelly, a very attractive thirty-something mother of three who has suffered with

Lyme for the last four years. "I know that sounds funny coming from a woman, but that tick took away from me more than just my good health and sanity. I can't tell you the problems it has caused between my husband and me. He kept thinking I was pushing him away, and I was trying to convince him that I was in *pain* and sex was the last thing on my mind.

"When he gave me an ultimatum, I finally told him if it was that important to him, go get 'it' someplace else and leave me alone. I don't think he did, but what's more shocking to me is that I actually said those words to him. I mean, I love my husband—he has always been my best friend and support. Sometimes I think I'm really going crazy and then I get depressed."

Patients report that not only do they tend to lose interest in sex, but that their sex lives also suffer as a result of the mood swings and verbal backlash that strain a close relationship. "A lot of what goes on under the sheets starts with the interaction and feelings that are generated when two people aren't anywhere near the bedroom," said one man. "You have someone who is going off the wall emotionally, being verbally abusive one minute and then critical or ultrasensitive the next—well, even if he *is* interested in sex, chances are his partner won't be because of hurt feelings and hostility. And that causes all kinds of problems as well."

As if all of this isn't enough to contend with, Lyme can both trigger and/or mask other psychological syndromes.

WHAT ELSE CAN POSSIBLY GO WRONG?

Laura was around ten years old when she contracted Lyme disease—her mother noticed a bull's-eye rash—but it took another three years to get a diagnosis. Besides having a severe headache for four and a half years, by the time she was fifteen she was displaying a whole host of compulsive behaviors. She would rip open all the new bars of soap. No towel or bedsheet felt clean enough and she changed clothes continually. She could never get anywhere on time because she had to check everything four times. She—and her family—feared she was going crazy.

Thirty-year-old Diane worked as an accountant at a large firm when she contracted Lyme while on vacation in California. By the time she was diagnosed eighteen months later, she could no longer function at her job. A normally easygoing person, she had become short-tempered and verbally abusive with everyone, could not sleep at night, had brief periods of blackout, and refused to go outdoors "where the ticks are." She was convinced that if she did not begin each day by reciting the alphabet, the Ten Commandments, and the names of the U.S. presidents in order, the day would be a disaster. Her father was on the verge of exploring mental institutions for his daughter when the antibiotics kicked in and the old Diane began to return.

Harry had been fighting Lyme for more than two years. Diagnosed late and displaying many neurological symptoms, he was under a doctor's care when his wife noticed that he was becoming obsessive about bugs. He'd look everywhere for them when he entered a room. He wouldn't sit in a chair until he had inspected it with a magnifying glass for ticks, and he meticulously checked all the food served to him, both at home and in restaurants, to the point of continuing to examine his food when everyone else was done.

Laura, Diane, and Harry were diagnosed separately as having obsessive-compulsive disorder (OCD), but treating doctors say they cannot honestly be sure whether the condition is caused directly by Lyme or whether the patients fall into the 2 to 3 percent of the population that suffers from this disorder naturally. It has been noticed, however, that the onset of OCD corresponds to other neurological aspects of Lyme in diagnosed patients, and seems to calm down as antibiotic treatment progresses.

Surely, it does not seem unreasonable that a person, after suffering with Lyme, becomes a little paranoid about checking for ticks. But OCD also precipitates weird thoughts that make no sense, says Dr. Fallon. These thoughts can be about anything from germs to sexually related situations to aggression.

Dr. Cary Hamlin has been treating an increasing number of Lyme patients with OCD in his office in rural Chester, New

Jersey. Board certified in psychiatry and neurology as well as psychopharmacology, Hamlin is highly published in journals and books and has made more than thirty professional presentations on anxiety disorders. He serves as an assistant professor of psychiatry at Columbia University and a peer reviewer for American Medical Informatics.

A tall man with a gentle voice, Hamlin has been at the cutting edge of utilizing computer technology to map the physiological changes in the brain caused by a number of disease agents and determining how those changes manifest as behavioral problems. He has no doubt that the Lyme spirochete causes havoc in the brain because he's seen the results.

"Lyme can definitely trigger OCD. Many infectious disease doctors will say, 'Okay, the patient is cured, so what's wrong with him?' The problem is that we're dealing with a significant anxiety disorder and how the nervous system is disordered is part of the drama in deciding how to fix it.

"How you fix the brain depends on how badly it's been injured," he says. "The main idea is to get rid of the Lyme and then deal with the damage it has done. Some neurological changes can be reversed, and we can measure through spectral analysis whether the left frontal lobe isn't talking to the right frontal lobe."

Hamlin says he has treated patients with everything from Tourette's syndrome to tic problems to a man whose morning ritual included speaking to his iguana in a certain way so the day could proceed. The issue is not just fear—like a fear of contamination—but anger and disgust mixed in. He has been working on a new neuro-feedback technique that addresses the mental disconnect Lyme disease patients suffer—a type of "weight lifting for the brain."

"There is no cookbook for this; nobody knows the recipe," says Hamlin. "The important thing to remember is that antibiotics are essential if the bug is still active and replicating. It's difficult to do anything to help the patient until you get rid of the bug."

Apart from true clinical depression, another psychological factor that is being mentioned in relation to Lyme disease is the "rage response." This is displayed primarily by males from adolescence to adulthood, and stories abound of fists being put through walls, heavy objects being lifted and thrown, and formerly docile people becoming enraged disproportionately to the given situation. Although sheer frustration over the other manifestations of the illness, the lack of diagnosis, and perhaps lack of immediate response to treatment would seem enough to provoke extreme anger, psychiatrists say that the cause could also be a temporal lobe seizure. This, like OCD, requires close scrutiny and evaluation by a psychiatrist.

Finally, at some point, most chronic Lyme patients get angry. This anger may be directed at the medical profession for not recognizing and treating the problem and thus preventing a chronic condition; it could be directed at those closest to them, for not being able to understand their pain or simply for being well; and it could be directed at themselves, for having the disease.

Scott has found an outlet for his anger—he brainstorms ideas for either curing Lyme or trying to work the bugs out of the current system of medical management: "When they finally find a cure for Lyme disease, I'm going to be so happy. And I'll be glad at that point that I had this experience, because I'll be stronger mentally and emotionally than other people. All of us will who have been through this. We've had to be to survive."

"A certain amount of anger is not all bad," says Fallon. "Everyone deals with it in a different way. Some intellectualize it, and some displace it. But everyone needs a support and information network where they can work this out of their systems. The bottom line is that you have to be your own advocate and search for your health—your physical and mental health."

The good news, he says, is that the last half-dozen or so years have brought a greater awareness among all branches of the medical profession as to how Lyme can affect the mental and emotional behavior of a victim.

The bad news is that, even with the advances that have been made, there are still many doctors in the field who are resistant to even considering Lyme as a cause of mental deterioration, and many social service agencies have not included the problems caused by Lyme in their protocols for service. This ignorance can result in the patient paying the ultimate price.

SUICIDE

Ingrid was a beautiful twenty-five-year-old who, despite a severe case of Lyme, managed to graduate from college and get accepted at a California law school. She worked with underprivileged children and struggled to stay on top of an illness that was gradually diminishing her health, her energy, and her financial resources.

As her health spiraled downward and her money evaporated, she sought help from various social service agencies. Social Security, Welfare, and Food Stamps all rejected her. At one point, she complained to her mother, she was told that in order to qualify for assistance, she had to be either under twenty-one, over sixty-five, pregnant, or a refugee.

Finally, on Christmas Eve 1994, Ingrid took her own life. Before she did, she sat in front of a video camera and made a tape recounting her struggle with Lyme disease. "I want people to understand what my life was like before Lyme, and how it fell apart after Lyme," she said on the tape. She recounted the isolation she felt, the deepening depression, and the eventual loss of memory and control over her life.

Unfortunately, Ingrid's story is being echoed across the country. Major depression ranks first among the causes of disability worldwide and more than 60 percent of people who die by suicide suffer from major depression, according to the American Foundation of Suicide Prevention's most recent numbers. Even more startling is this: a person dies by suicide about every eighteen minutes in the United States. An attempt is made an estimated once a minute. Suicide is this country's eleventh leading cause of death, with depression being the most prominent catalyst. A high percentage of Lyme patients—particularly those who are chronically ill—suffer some form of depression, and this is not a symptom to be easily dismissed.

Lyme support group leaders and advocates are concerned about the growing numbers of both official and unofficial suicides attributed to Lyme disease. While no solid numbers exist, people like Stephen Nostrom, founder of the Lyme Borrelia Outreach Foundation in Mattituck, New York, and Marvina Lodge, president of the Florida Lyme Disease Network in Zellwood, Florida, are becoming all too familiar with those urgent cries for help.

"I've literally had calls in the middle of the night with someone saying, 'I've got a twenty-gauge shotgun and a fifth of whisky and tonight's the night,'" says Nostrom, who was diagnosed with Lyme in 1987 and hosted a monthly cable television show on Lyme disease. "I've had calls from telephone booths, at all hours of the day and night—I even tracked down one teenage girl who had called and left messages. We found her down by the water."

Lodge agrees. "What complicates things even further is when the Lyme patient, who is feeling ill and frightened in the first place, then has to fight on all fronts just so someone will believe him or her, let alone address the problem and begin treatment. It's easy for depression to take over. Way too easy."

Physicians and family members alike need to be aware that disseminated cases of Lyme disease do include a psychiatric component that, if unrecognized and/or ignored, could result in the Lyme sufferer's depression and despair reaching levels where the only thought is to end the pain . . . by whatever means available.

COPING AND SURVIVING

Dr. Richard Goldman, a veterinarian who has struggled back from the brink of blindness and despondency with Lyme, says, "Patience is not a virtue—it's a survival tool if you have Lyme disease!" Although it is difficult to infuse someone else with patience, Kathy Cavert, an R.N. with Lyme, who founded the

Midwest Lyme Disease Association and published *LymeAid* out of Independence, Missouri, used her extensive psychological training and experience to offer some practical coping skills to Lyme patients. Ranging from the physical to the spiritual, Kathy's tips can be condensed to the mnemonic FACE PEG:

Flexibility   Also called "rolling with the punches." Lyme patients must recognize that rigid rules of life need to be set aside if they are going to cope successfully and win out over this relapsing and remitting disease.

Awareness   Not only of one's mortality but of the choice one has to make whether to rely on external sources for satisfaction or on internal sources. "This is referred to as the external locus of control versus the internal," says Kathy. "The internal control is very powerful as we depend upon our own strengths and resources to stay afloat. We can be sorely disappointed if we let our external environment control our feelings."

Counseling   Essential for those who are dealing with physical and emotional problems prior to contracting Lyme, counseling is also an emotional handrail for those who are feeling their way through this confusing and frustrating illness. The need for reassurance is great and short-term counseling has been proven to be of great benefit in marshaling a person's internal resources and reducing depression.

Education   The disease becomes much less mysterious when one makes an effort to understand the clinical symptoms and signs. In addition, a Lyme patient must be a vigilant medical consumer in order to obtain the best care available and not be led astray by agencies or doctors who are unaware.

Pacing   This is a way of saving energy, preventing overfatigue and possible injury, and being able to live as normal a life as possible. Lyme patients may have to realize that while they have an active case of Lyme they may not be able to work as many hours, stay out as late, or even accomplish the same number of tasks in a day as they did prior to Lyme.

Exercise Increasingly, knowledgeable doctors are recommending regular regimens of aerobic exercise for their Lyme patients, even if that means following a brief exercise period with a nap. Not only does exercise raise the body temperature and suppress some of the more bothersome symptoms, it is good therapy for the mind as well. In fact, even those Lyme patients who have difficulty with the arthritic component of the disease report that strenuous physical exercise makes them feel better.

Giving It is easy to fall into the pit of self-absorption. After all, with the plethora of aches and pains and lifestyle changes Lyme may inflict, the tendency for preoccupation with one's own health looms large. To get on with life and put those pains in perspective, get out of the house, call a friend, volunteer some time answering the telephone at a literacy program—do something to remind yourself that a lot of other people out there need help too.

Finally, have faith—in the fact that you are not alone in this illness, in the fact that there are many people who are waging the battle against Lyme, and in yourself. You are not going crazy; you just have Lyme disease.

Having faith is admittedly more difficult for a patient when a doctor misses the diagnosis. It is equally difficult for a doctor when the government or a public health department refuses to validate his or her diagnosis. Both doctors and patients are recognizing that despite the growing recognition of Lyme disease, it is still a political football.

7.

The Politics of Diagnosing Lyme Disease

Note the following:

■ Missouri—In the spring of 1994, a nationally renowned Lyme disease pioneer was approached by the CDC to cooperate in a study to dispute his contention that the illness was running rampant in the Midwest. After cooperating fully and documenting the outstanding evidence—the CDC documented even *more* cases of Lyme than had this physician—the doctor was asked to sign off on the printed results, which bore thirty-two pages of errors, misinformation, and false statements. Both he and a state health official refused to sign, due to the mistruths. They were told that the report would be published with or without their signatures. The physician retained all of his records, proving the false report. During the summer of 1996, the CDC conceded that a "Lyme-like illness" existed in Missouri, and in 2002 finally called the illness Master's disease, after the physician who had spent a decade documenting and successfully treating what is called Lyme in the rest of the country.

■ Detroit—In 2003, the laboratory of a professor emeritus at Wayne State University was invaded by state marshals with handcuffs. She was threatened with jail and an exorbitant fine. Her crime? She had refined a test that was successfully identifying and documenting the *Borrelia burgdorferi* spirochete in blood samples, a test that had been published and well received in a European medical journal. "I had to agree not to help doctors diagnose and treat Lyme disease or go to jail," she says indignantly. "Can you imagine being treated like that in this day and age in the United States of America?"

▪ Florida—The official standpoint of the Department of Health is that Lyme disease does not exist in this tourist-oriented playground. Yet a Gainesville veterinarian, who came close to losing his eyesight and his practice because of Lyme, counsels hundreds of callers per month who are beset by the classic symptoms. And in Miami, a mother is reported as having Munchausen by Proxy, that is, when a parent deliberately induces a child's illness for the attention and sympathy it elicits, by a resident physician who knows little about Lyme disease but was disturbed at the numerous medical symptoms the mother listed over a number of visits. Her child had previously tested positive for Lyme, a fact ignored by the doctor.

▪ Between 1995 and 2002, more than thirty respected and, in some cases published and peer-reviewed, physicians who have been at the forefront of diagnosing, treating, and documenting Lyme disease had their practices and offices invaded by state medical boards, spurred by "anonymous tips," and were forced to spend months and thousands of dollars defending themselves, their licenses, and their integrity against harassment and, in many cases, unsubstantiated lies.

Since the original *Coping with Lyme Disease* was compiled ten years ago, the political face of Lyme disease has only gotten uglier. The numbers continue to skyrocket; there have been more restrictive changes in drug management and treatment protocols; and scientific findings continue to reveal a portrait of an organism so virulent in its ability to mutate and evade antibiotics that many physicians—under the threat of having their licenses lifted by state medical boards for "overtreating Lyme"—have thrown up their hands in frustration.

In an age of miracle drugs, instant gratification, and global technology, it is difficult to believe that so many people who are sick from the bite of a tick are unable to get a simple prescription for antibiotics that will take care of the problem. This should be easy, right? After all, doctors have routinely prescribed antibiotics for teenage acne for a couple of years without thinking twice. Why is Lyme disease so difficult? Why is it so political? And why has it so divided medical professionals?

The simple answer is money.

To many clinicians and patients across the country, the politics of diagnosing Lyme disease is similar to the politics surrounding the acknowledgment of another monumental hazard, albeit fictional.

When the great white shark of *Jaws* fame relentlessly feasted on unsuspecting bathers off the shores of the fictional town of Amity, the reactions ranged from the hysteria of those who saw sharks in every ripple of the water's surface to denial by the town fathers that anything unusual had occurred. The official thinking went: If we don't acknowledge the shark, the tourists won't stay away and we won't have a problem. But of course, the shark kept attacking and the ensuing panic and death toll turned out to be worse than if the authorities had simply acknowledged and addressed the problem. Today, we are suffering from that same "Amity mentality," but the shark is Lyme disease, and the consequences are not fictional.

From California to Tennessee and Texas to Florida, Lyme disease sufferers have been forced to travel hundreds of miles—often out of state—on a regular basis for treatment because of medical ignorance and hostility or the governmental fear that acknowledging Lyme disease would be injurious to the economic vitality of an area. The prevailing "Amity-speak" at work here is: If we don't acknowledge Lyme disease, then doctors won't look for it, so there will be no Lyme disease.

But, of course, Lyme disease does exist, and this roadblock to immediate and efficient health care has inspired a groundswell of medical consumer activism paralleling the early AIDS demonstrations, networks, confrontations, and legislation.

Like AIDS and some forms of cancer, the treatment of chronic Lyme disease—which has finally been acknowledged by the CDC and is the subject of a national study (see chapter 15)—can be expensive and sometimes controversial. In addition, its comparison to another relapsing and remitting spiro-chetal illness—syphilis—inspires a negative attitude among medical representatives because the disease does not respond to the officially endorsed treatment. Additionally, many academics, institutions, and commercial companies have cut deals for grants or product manufacturing that would suffer if an independent researcher should come up with a "gold standard" test or cure. And finally, city fathers view it negatively because this is an infection borne not by an individual's behavior but by environ-mental agents, and *nobody* wants to be "blamed" for a hazard.

The irony is that, the way Lyme disease is spreading, the question of where one acquired it will be moot. The focus needs to be on who is going to provide the most efficient diagnosis and treatment before growing numbers of debilitated citizens are denied the chance to live normal lives.

REPORTING = LOOKING = REPORTING

Like most nine-year-olds, Mandy loved Halloween. She espe-cially looked forward to her trip to the local pumpkin farm to pick out just the right one for her family's jack-o'-lantern.

After a trip to the pumpkin farm in 1988 however, she devel-oped a rash. Her mother informed doctors about the rash but was told not to worry, as rashes are a common and minor affliction in rural New Jersey. Then came a series of increasing complaints of blistering headaches, painful joints, and other symptoms from the young girl, who was normally outgoing, friendly, and active. After six months of increasing debilitation, Mandy slipped into a coma. Her mother begged the doctors to administer a Lyme test. They refused, brushing her off with denials of Lyme dis-ease's existence. Mandy's mother didn't give up.

Finally, when the little girl came out of the coma, the Lyme test was given. Mandy was positive, but antibiotics prolonged her life for only eighteen months. Mandy died because of swelling of her brain due to Lyme disease. Hers was a death that could have been avoided.

"Somebody should have said, 'Let's try antibiotics at this time,' but they were too busy telling us it wasn't Lyme," said Mandy's mother in an article for the *Trentonian* newspaper.

Some may argue that not much was known about Lyme disease back in 1988, that what happened to Mandy would not happen today. Unfortunately, nothing is further from the truth. Despite the fact that the CDC has been tracking Lyme for fifteen years and that there has been a recent "discovery" of Lyme by both public health officials and the media, this disease is still in its infancy in terms of our understanding of how it operates, how to get rid of it, and how to educate both the public and those who have the power to help eradicate it.

"Our job is to protect the public health—disease prevention and control," said Dr. David Dennis, director of the CDC Lyme Disease Project, in operation since 1989. "The problem is, with Lyme disease we don't have a proper tool at the present time to say 'Yes, this is definitely Lyme' or 'No, this definitely is not Lyme.'"

The current case definition of Lyme disease has undergone several revolutions, with the final interpretation being the most restrictive and limiting. This description is admittedly bare-bones, according to Dennis, and leaves out many of the variations that Lyme disease includes. For this reason, the CDC warns doctors and insurance companies repeatedly not to use its case definition for diagnostic and evaluation purposes.

To fit the CDC's Lyme disease national surveillance case definition, a patient must have one of the following:

1. A physician-diagnosed EM rash of at least 5 cm in diameter, or
2. Laboratory confirmation of exposure to *B. burgdorferi* by two tests and at least one systemic manifestation.

As was previously stated, however, not everyone gets or remembers a rash, and the current serologic tests have been unreliable. Using only these two criteria to describe Lyme is like having every town report how many apples it has, with the definition of apples being only that they are solid red in color and have a diameter of three inches.

"The diagnosis of Lyme disease has to be a clinical diagnosis," emphasized Dennis, "meaning that doctors should use the tests as just another tool when considering a diagnosis of Lyme. For tracking purposes, we have to make sure each case is exactly alike, even if that represents only a small number. But we encourage doctors to report *all* cases of Lyme disease to their health departments. Many states have a two-drawer system; one drawer for the ones that fit our strict criteria, and one for all the others. But none of that works if we can't get doctors to report it."

The Lyme disease case report is a simple, one-page, twenty-five-question form. Why don't doctors report? Like the disease, the answers can be complicated.

There are always those doctors who retort: "It takes too much time" and "I hate doing paperwork."

There are a good number who are frustrated at attempting to report cases of Lyme disease; if a case does not match the CDC criteria, it is refused by the health department. Runarounds at various health departments, according to doctors surveyed, also include being put on "hold" when mentioning Lyme disease, being told that nobody there is assigned to handle Lyme, and being referred from clerk to clerk until the telephone is disconnected.

There are also doctors, such as those in the hyperendemic section of southern New Jersey, who are threatened by insurance companies and medical boards for overreporting Lyme disease. As was explained in the *Asbury Park Press,* doctors who reported large numbers of Lyme disease cases would be in danger of having their medical licenses lifted pending an investigation. This type of scare tactic levied by the larger insurance carriers tends to motivate doctors to refer suspected Lyme cases to other physicians rather than diagnose, report, and treat.

All of the above factors lead many physicians to stop short of reporting Lyme, concluding: "It really doesn't matter anyway."

They are wrong. Reporting Lyme disease *does* matter.

Underreporting of a disease leads to more "Amity-speak": If we underreport, then there is no problem, so there is no need for funding to find a cure for a problem that does not exist.

Underreporting matters to patients like Lillith, in South Carolina, who began having to travel to New Jersey for Lyme treatment when her own doctor, bowing to pressure from his partners, told her that after two months of treatment she "should be cured of a disease that doesn't really affect the Carolinas anyway."

It matters to patients like fourteen-year-old Corey, who went from being an achiever both on and off the basketball court to being unable to walk across a room without trembling and tripping, and whose New York doctor refused to see him when his mother called to report the rash and other symptoms, stating, "This Lyme disease is just a bunch of hysteria. Don't worry about it." Corey now has permanent damage to his brain and his heart as a result of a late diagnosis.

Reporting the disease matters to health departments, both in endemic states like Rhode Island, Wisconsin, and New Jersey and in those other states where Lyme is spreading like wildfire and is competing for public health dollars with AIDS, tuberculosis, and other infectious diseases. Reporting also serves to remind health departments that ticks cannot read state border signs, and that they continually cross into areas where they "are not supposed to be."

And it matters to those doctors who are running themselves into the ground treating Lyme patients in the face of suspicion and criticism from academic circles and many peers who have fallen victim to the prevailing "Amity-speak."

TRACKING A LYME-LIKE ILLNESS

Mark Twain would have been comfortable in Cape Girardeau, Missouri. Perched on the banks of the Mississippi River, the town provides its farmers and friendly residents a view clear across to Illinois and, on an inspired day, maybe even to Kentucky. These are hardworking people who don't stop to complain about little aches and pains, and certainly not rashes, as they toil during the week to put food on the table and enjoy the small-town life with their families on the weekends.

Dr. Edwin Masters, of Cape Girardeau, describes himself as a "simple country doc," but his quick grin and folksy homilies can't hide his acuity and concern when discussing the nearly one thousand cases of the disease he has diagnosed but cannot get his state to recognize.

"I'm a tree farmer by avocation, so when the state medical society was holding a conference, they asked me to prepare a talk on Lyme disease. Hell, I didn't know anything about Lyme, and I didn't believe it existed in these parts, but I operate on Masters's Maxim—that is, anything that's worth doing is worth overdoing. I collected hundreds of articles, prepared slides, studied, and presented my findings at the meeting."

That was the beginning of a five-year crusade, but the major obstacle was the fact that the *Ixodes dammini* tick, the primary Lyme vector, was not common in Missouri.

"Suddenly, certain illnesses and symptoms I had been seeing began falling into place," said Masters. "I had patients who came in with these look-alike bull's-eye rashes, and look-alike spirochetes, and look-alike symptoms, so I made look-alike diagnoses. But when I questioned them about tick bites, the ticks they described were often the size of a watermelon seed with a white spot in the middle. I was the most skeptical of all, but these were farmers, school kids, old ladies, laborers—people who wouldn't know an *Amblyomma americanum* [Lone Star tick] from Godzilla, yet they were all describing the same thing! I thought, 'How can this be?'"

Continuing to operate on Masters's Maxim, he discovered that Missouri is directly in the path of one of the greatest flyways in the country, where millions of migratory birds land in their treks from north to south and back again. Not only were the birds pausing to refresh themselves in Missouri, they apparently were also depositing infected ticks along their migratory path.

Masters meticulously photographs and cultures his patients'

rashes, and he also keeps both blood and urine samples on all of his suspected Lyme disease cases. Until the CDC established that in Missouri the Lyme spirochete was carried not by the *Ixodes* tick but by others (and named the illness Masters had been documenting Master's disease), a lot of patients fell through the cracks.

"And those cracks extend from Indiana to Nebraska and Iowa to Texas," said Masters. "I'm a country doc in a small town and I have to see these suffering patients. I can't give them two weeks of whatever treatment, then close my eyes and say, 'You are cured. Go away. Go see a psychiatrist and don't bug me.' I have to live with these people, and they come back! I have to call it like I see it. These people are sick, and they deserve to be treated."

The Missouri story is not dissimilar to the situations found in states from Tennessee and Kentucky to Alabama and Florida and the Virginias. Again, patients were turning up in droves with classic Lyme symptoms but being turned away by doctors who had been told the disease did not exist outside of the Northeast. This contradiction came to the attention of Southeast Outdoor Press Association (SEOPA) members, whose professional and recreational lives revolve around the enjoyment of outdoor sports, including hunting, fishing, camping, and hiking. Not only were these men and women struggling to bring the tick-borne disease to the public's and the medical profession's attention—by filing numerous stories on this illness contracted by those who worked out-of-doors, such as farmers, utility workers, and parks and landscape professionals—many of the press members themselves began falling victim to Lyme disease. The result was the creation of a specially organized effort.

"Last year in South Carolina, SEOPA decided to take a more activist part in educating people about Lyme disease," said Norris Blackburn, a resident of Morristown, Tennessee, and a former SEOPA president. "We need to educate physicians as well as the public because doctors are seeing more of this than ever before, but aren't recognizing it until the patient slips into the late or chronic stage and is affected for life. We are going to be staging major efforts to being the true facts about Lyme disease to the attention of the medical profession and urge that something be done."

Part of that "something" revolves around documentation of vectors and levels of infection in a specific geographic area, to gain the CDC's acknowledgment of a Lyme disease problem in that area. This type of painstaking work began as an intriguing intellectual exercise for Dr. James Oliver, professor of biology and director of arthropodology and parisitology for Georgia Southern University. Like Masters, however, Dr. Oliver is now a passionate laborer in the Lyme disease field, after witnessing the unrelenting pain and suffering that was going unheeded.

"The CDC is conservative, and rightly so, because they don't want a panic developing, but people with increasing symptoms are becoming distraught. This is such a diffuse issue: we have the awareness versus unawareness and the need for research-type studies. The problem with getting study participants is, when a patient is ill and goes to his doctor, the doctor can say, 'Well, I think this is Lyme disease and I can prescribe an antibiotic to start you getting well, or we can enroll you in this study and over the course of the next twelve to twenty-four weeks your symptoms will be studied and some of you will be given antibiotics.' Which way do you think the patient is going to go?"

Another problem in Georgia, as in Missouri, is that the Lyme-carrying *Ixodes* tick was rare, despite the increasing number of Lyme cases. So Oliver meticulously documented, by DNA-sequencing probes, that the infected black-legged tick was the same as the *Ixodes,* isolating it in four large geographic locations from the northern part of Georgia to Cape Canaveral in Florida. His research was presented at the Fifth International Conference on Lyme Disease, sponsored by the NIH, thus opening the door for official recognition of the disease. This is still slow in coming.

"I think we have to go with the caveat that with all we still don't know about Lyme disease, maybe all the last *i*'s aren't dotted when people are suffering but we still need to treat them. Sure, we may actually be treating a few people who don't have it, but is that worse than missing the many who are suffering and sliding into chronic illness? I don't think so."

This is a sentiment expressed by many who are in the midst of the Lyme battle, but it is not one eagerly embraced by the medical profession overall. At least, not among the more vocal conservatives.

THE POLITICS OF THE MEDICAL PROFESSION

During the mid-1970s, hospitals across the country were seeing thousands of patients complaining of extreme stomach pain, many of them in such pain that they couldn't function. Surgery was commonplace. Then, a drug named Tagamet was discovered. Upon being administered, this drug relieved the stomach distress, and surgery rates dropped. It was a dramatic discovery, and soon Tagamet became the number one prescribed drug in the country, with patients actively seeking it out.

However, doctors were told that they could prescribe Tagamet for only two weeks, or they would be considered "cowboys" or wild doctors. The patients, sliding back into pain and dysfunction, continued seeking out new doctors to prescribe the drug so they could continue with their lives. Fifteen years later, medical science decided that the patients were right all along, and now doctors routinely prescribe Tagamet for prolonged periods of time.

This particular case illustrates the slowness with which the medical profession, rightly cautious, moves, as well as how it can ignore evidence to the detriment of patients for a long period of time.

The politics of Lyme includes some interesting facts:

■ Unlike the case with other diseases, such as cancer, the diagnosis of Lyme depends on whether or not the doctor in question agrees with certain treatment protocols.

▪ Unlike the case with other diseases, the "cure" is defined in terms of how many antibiotics have been administered and for what length of time, rather than cessation of symptoms and absence of infection.

▪ Unlike the case with other diseases, the question of a Lyme diagnosis often rests solely upon the doctor's ability to make a clinical diagnosis (a return to the "old days" of medicine), instead of a reliance on empirical tests. Contemporary doctors are not trained for this and, in fact, are discouraged from trusting their clinical acumen.

▪ For any or all of the above reasons, Lyme diagnosis and treatment have caused medical professionals to take up arms against each other, each publicly hurling aspersions against the others' credibility and practices. These verbal attacks have been fired primarily from the purely academic researchers toward the clinician researchers and practitioners, whose work has been dismissed as "anecdotal" and "junk science."

Is this just another example of the age-old competition between the academicians, who enjoy the luxury of being more conservative because they are not dealing with patients daily, and the doctors in the trenches, who must treat sufferer after sufferer? Is it the snobbery of those who consider themselves "pure scientists" versus the "cowboys in the field" whose research may be privately funded? Perhaps. There is also the criticism that those associated with government and academic institutions must maintain lengthy time lines in research procedure in order to justify the much-needed allocations they receive.

All three points can be argued, and many of the more vociferous opponents on both sides suffer from what author Peter Senge, in his book *The Fifth Discipline,* calls one of the modern-day organizational learning disabilities: the "I am my position" identity, where a person stakes out a territory, identifies with it, and then defends it to the death—even in the face of contradictory evidence.

With Lyme disease, however, there is another factor involved. Because of the diversity of the disease and the lack of reliable empirical data, there is a great fear of personal liability.

FAULT, LIABILITY, AND RESPONSIBILITY

In a special exhibit presented at the National Museum of Health and Medicine in Washington, D.C., in November 1992, the question of medical ethics as it relates to human values and the complicity of doctors in Nazi experiments were highlighted. Entitled "The Value of the Human Being: Medicine in Germany, 1918–1945," the exhibit disturbed many in both the medical and the lay communities. The viewpoint was presented that during World War II, many doctors became agents of the state instead of advocates of the patient; they began viewing people as impersonal research statistics instead of individuals.

The exhibit further maintained that by joining the Nazi party, more than thirty-eight thousand doctors and scientists (almost half of Germany's total) were allowed to get research grants, receive promotions at universities, and take over the practices of the thousands of Jews who were no longer allowed to practice medicine.

The exhibit prompted Dr. James S. Todd, executive vice president of the American Medical Association, to comment in a *New York Times* article: "One of our biggest challenges today is balancing medicine and health against the resources available. But we have to strive to do this without forgetting about the patients we serve." Doctors, he said, have a special responsibility because people entrust them with their privacy as well as with their lives.

The politics of Lyme disease today can be likened somewhat to the mind-set of probably well-meaning physicians who got swept up in the Nazi regime. Struggling to support their families, continue their research, and maintain their career tracks, many unwittingly acted in passive complicity toward the deaths of millions.

Some may think this is too strong a statement—a totally inappropriate analogy. Yet when the most trusted professionals in a country—physicians—opt for reducing people and suffering to statistics because it allows them to comfortably maintain the status quo, as opposed to placing themselves and perhaps their careers on the line to relieve human suffering, isn't that reducing the value of a human being?

This is exactly what happens when a doctor refuses to listen to evidence of a disease—be it Lyme, AIDS, or cancer—because to diagnose and treat it might open him or her to question. This is exactly what happens when doctors who live in high-end suburban neighborhoods fight any acknowledgment of Lyme disease in their areas because they are afraid of their real estate values going down. And this is exactly what happens when otherwise bright and sincere doctors refuse to accept documentation of disease that is contrary to their "I am my position" stand, because to do so would mean admitting fallibility, even when human suffering is at stake.

I don't want to fall into the pit of indicting *all* doctors. There are many, many out there, God bless them, who do listen, and who do act as advocates for their patients at the risk of being considered out of the "mainstream." These men and women are true healers. Lyme disease, however, has caused many more to avoid some sticky issues, and sitting on the fence can cause a delay in diagnosis and therefore in treatment and possible eradication early on.

Another factor preventing doctors from dealing with Lyme is that we live in a litigious society. One cannot fault doctors for being cautious. It is also recognized that the practice of medicine is an *art* and not an exact science. But the "Amity-speak" at work here is: If I diagnose Lyme, I have to treat. If I treat and the patient doesn't respond well (or my peers object), I could be in trouble. Therefore, I won't diagnose.

This, unfortunately, is not an unusual position. And the one who pays is the patient, who can slip from a curable state into a debilitated and chronic condition.

INFORMED CONSENT AGREEMENTS

To respond to ailing patients with diffuse and Lyme-suspicious complaints, yet attempt to protect themselves, some doctors who treat the disease are taking a page out of the surgeon's guidebook and drawing up "informed consent" agreements.

Although viewed as impractical for a "normal" doctor-patient relationship, the informed consent agreement can be useful when dealing with a disease and treatment protocol that carry some controversy, according to Stephen Sepaniak, an attorney specializing in health and medicine in Lyme-endemic Morristown, New Jersey. And, if it encourages more doctors to deal with Lyme disease, such an agreement should be considered.

"One of the greatest areas of dispute between patients and physicians has to do with whether the physician disclosed to the patient all the risks of treatment, alternative forms of treatment, and even the risks of nontreatment. Clearly, these should be discussed," said Sepaniak. "When there are controversies surrounding treatment, as in Lyme disease, if I were a physician, I would spend a substantial amount of time discussing the different forms of treatment—reviewing the pros and cons of each regimen, and why one may be more appropriate than another. Only then would I give a patient my recommendation for a course of treatment and my reasons for that recommendation."

Some overcautious doctors videotape entire discussions and the patient's consent, but a written form is more standard. The paragraphs should include the benefits of the treatment, the risks, the alternative forms of treatment, and the risks of non-treatment. Then, the physician should outline his proposed course of action, with possible side effects, and sign the form, along with the patient.

"If a physician treats a patient negligently, he or she is still liable and no informed consent is going to provide blanket immunity," said Sepaniak, but the act of using an informed consent form forces the doctor to sit down and discuss, at length, the illness and the course of action. It takes some time, but it is a necessary expenditure of time that will benefit both the patient and the physician.

Educating and winning the proper attention of the country's populace is an important battle in the politics of diagnosing and treating Lyme. One would think that the education would come from the medical profession, but again, as with AIDS, it is the mass of Lyme sufferers and their loved ones who are leading the fight for recognition and treatment.

A GRASSROOTS MOVEMENT

Eighteen years ago, when Pat Smith was on the board of education for Wall Township, New Jersey, a strange illness began attacking teachers and students alike. No one, it seemed, had any information on this strange thing called Lyme disease that had put a number of them in the hospital in critical condition. Pat found out that the only information available was from Earl Naval Weapons Station, because they had already experienced fifty-six cases of this debilitating illness, so she took what they had to give, did some research, and began to inform her local community.

Within the next few years, both of Pat's daughters contracted Lyme and her family was plunged into the depths of Lyme hell. Bounced from doctor to doctor, fighting for a diagnosis and then fighting for treatment, Pat watched her scholarly and athletic teenage daughters begin to shake with grand mal seizures and experience hallucinations coupled with incredible bodily pain. There was a time when she couldn't leave the house for three months because one daughter's fear and pain were so great. "The night that I came home to a dark house and found her in a fetal position, unable to speak, I promised that if she ever recovered from this, I would never let another parent go through this on their own."

Her daughters gradually recovered through the use of long-term antibiotics and went on to graduate from college and lead productive lives. And Pat never forgot the promise she uttered out of a mother's anguish.

Today, after forming the first New Jersey Lyme Committee and serving on the Governor's Commission on Lyme Disease, Pat heads the Lyme Disease Association (LDA), which has united a number of state affiliates under a national umbrella and provided more than one million research dollars to twenty-eight different projects ranging from genetic and serology studies to those involving the underdiagnosis and effects of Lyme in women and children. The LDA (together with the Lyme Disease Foundation) was instrumental in bringing accurate information on the faulty and injurious Lyme vaccine to the FDA's attention. The LDA has also served as the catalyst for a host of federal legislation, national public education programs, and the production of books, guides, and videotapes for educating school systems, medical professionals, and the public about Lyme disease.

LDA headquarters is still Smith's home; there are no paid employees, including herself, so all funds raised go directly to research and education. She works nearly round-the-clock, fielding phone calls from sources as disparate as the U.S. Senate, a European research hospital, a Tel Aviv physician, a Hollywood set designer, and a frightened mother in Kansas who can't get a definitive diagnosis for her son. She is driven by the thousands of sick people and the memories of her own sick girls. "People are finally beginning to feel as though they are part of a larger cause," says Smith. "That's the way it has to work in order to effect a difference."

The story of the LDA's genesis is duplicated across the country. Faced with rejection, ignorance, and lack of treatment, men and women whose lives have been infected with Lyme become warriors in a battle for education and treatment. Some even leave their original professions behind in their fight for others' benefit.

The Ukiah, California-based Lyme Disease Resource Center (LDRC) was begun by Phyllis Mervine, who also founded and published the first national Lyme disease informational newsletter, *The Lyme Times,* following her own struggle with the disease in the late 1980s. Today the LDRC keeps abreast of the constantly changing Lyme climate and disseminates information on its website (see appendix C). The battle continues, as many doctors avoid putting themselves in a position of having to treat

Lyme patients—and deal with the potential diagnostic and political baggage that entails—by continuing to maintain that "patients are hysterical and Lyme is easy to diagnose and cure," Mervine says. "I was told by one doctor that 'It is not our job to put our livelihoods on the line for our patients.' But isn't that a question involving the Hippocratic Oath?"

Mervine says that in order to combat the "head in the sand" mentality prevalent in much of California, her organization is in the process of compiling hard data to support legislation that would require laboratories to report Lyme test results directly to the CDC. She is certain that this will help raise the red flag so physicians will have to look for, and deal with, Lyme disease in their own backyards.

Time For Lyme, founded in 1998 under the name Greenwich Lyme Disease Task Force by Debbie Siciliano and Diane Blanchard—two mothers whose children and families were being devastated by Lyme disease—has focused on endowing the first national research center for the study of Lyme and other tick-borne illnesses at Columbia University. They have also created a prototype tick removal kit that is not only being used by the Connecticut Red Cross, but is in demand at school districts and Red Cross affiliates across the country.

The Lyme Disease Foundation was begun by businesswoman Karen Forschner, who contracted Lyme during her pregnancy with her son, Jamie. He was infected with the disease through the placenta and died after kindergarten from a series of malformations and complications arising from it. The foundation, run by Karen and her husband, Tom, has been responsible for international conferences, legislation, and continuing research and education on various aspects of the disease.

The Lyme Disease Network, based in East Brunswick, New Jersey, was begun by Carol and Bill Stolow after their three young daughters came down with Lyme and they had to fight for treatment on their behalf. Initially operating a hotline and educational service only in their home state, the network now helps coordinate information on the Internet for support groups, doctors, researchers, and patients across the country, and provides an information line for doctors wishing to find out more about the disease.

For all of these groups, and many more notwithstanding, the recognition of Lyme disease as a potentially dangerous and debilitating illness begins with a recognition and acknowledgment that a problem does exist—as is illustrated by one of Dr. Masters's mental exercises. "Look around the room and for fifteen seconds memorize everything that's red," he says. "Now close your eyes. Tell me everything you saw in the room that was green. Chances are, you won't remember a thing. The eye only sees what the mind lets it. We have to let doctors realize that Lyme disease is out there so we can do something about it."

Recognition of Lyme begins with the symptoms, as varied and subjective as they may be, and then knowing where to go for help.

II.

SPECIAL AGES,

SPECIAL

PROBLEMS

Knowledge is little; to know the right context is much; to know the right spot is everything.

—HUGO VON HOFMANNSTHAL,
AUSTRIAN POET AND PLAYWRIGHT

8.

The Young Child

Two-year-old Tommy had been considered mentally retarded almost since infancy. When a new pediatrician grew suspicious of this diagnosis during a patient history session with the parents, he ordered a new set of tests. Tommy's parents were both horrified and pleasantly stunned to find out that their son had Lyme disease, probably contracted when he was six months old and on a family vacation. After a course of aggressive antibiotic therapy, Tommy rebounded like the normal two-year-old he was.

Eight-year-old Jackie drove her teachers crazy with complaints. She had stomachaches, headaches, conjunctivitis, nausea, joint pain, blurry vision, and difficulty sitting still in class. The school nurse finally told her parents that they should consider psychological help for their obviously disturbed child. Four months and three doctors later, Jackie was diagnosed with Lyme disease and placed on antibiotics. Eighteen months later, she is on the soccer team, enjoys playing the piano, and is consistently on the honor roll.

Ten-year-old Jenna's Lyme disease followed a cycle similar to Jackie's, but she also lost the use of her right hand and arm. It took six months and five doctors before her parents found a doctor who believed that Jenna's symptoms had an organic, not a psychological, base, and who searched for the diagnosis. One evening, in the midst of a myriad of interviews and invasive tests, Jenna presented herself to her parents and tearfully cried, "I know what's wrong; I have AIDS and you just don't want to tell me!"

Fifty percent of all reported Lyme disease cases involve children under the age of twelve. Of that group, the largest percentage of victims are between the ages of one and five. If adults find respectful diagnosis and treatment difficult to obtain, they are even more elusive for young children who are dependent upon the adults in their world to listen, believe, understand, and then serve as tenacious advocates for them.

Some of the special challenges to diagnosing children ranging in age from infancy to eleven years old include:

■ *They don't realize what is "normal."* Unlike adults, who have a track record of wellness, children, with their limited history and experience, may not even realize that everyone else walks around free of headache or of other symptoms that come and go.

■ *They cannot always articulate symptoms.* This is particularly true in the prelanguage child, who must rely on the observations of the adults around him or her and their knowledge as to what is normal. Because so many children are also in daycare situations, there is a reliance on these caretakers to observe and note changes. Even the school-age child may have difficulty articulating a pain that waxes and wanes, periods of fatigue, or sensitivity to sound or touch.

■ *They cannot remember sequences.* Children's frames of reference are such that if a hurt goes away they brush it from their minds and get on with life. If the pain returns, they may not be able to remember any sequential information that might provide some clue as to the pain's cause.

■ *Getting someone to listen.* If adults find this aspect of disease reporting difficult, pity the poor child, who must compete in the adult world for attention to a stomachache, weak ankles, tingling in the fingers or face ("My face feels funny," said one little girl repeatedly to her dad. "Your face *looks* funny," he would lovingly reply. Unfortunately, she was trying to tell him she was feeling tingling—a neurological symptom), and changes in sleep or personal patterns. (How many well-meaning parents crack down on television watching, play activities, and snacks when confronted with a child who complains that he can't sleep at night, has diarrhea, or is tired in school?)

• *Being believed.* More often than not, the children who complain of a kaleidoscope of aches are told they have growing pains, are just trying to get attention, are attempting to get out of school/homework/chores, are malingering, or simply are faking it.

In the popular movie *Ferris Bueller's Day Off,* the following advice is sagely given: "Don't overfake; it will get you a trip to the pediatrician and that's worse!" Dr. Louis Corsaro, a pediatrician and father of eight who practices in the hyperendemic area of Westchester County, New York, firmly believes the film's advice mirrors reality, and that more parents, teachers, and doctors need to listen to the young child who is attempting to convey a message of illness, particularly if something like Lyme disease is a possibility.

"Children don't lie when it comes to aches and pains, and they don't exaggerate," he said. "It should be easy to tell when a child is really ill because they only have two speeds—sleep and fast. As a pediatrician in an area where I've handled hundreds and hundreds of children with Lyme, about a third of them with chronic Lyme, there is no question in my mind that if a diagnosis is made early, short-term antibiotics are effective. But if children are dismissed as complainers, if there is a delay in focusing on the symptoms that are being presented—particularly if one is living in an area where Lyme is endemic—the child can go into a chronic stage, which is much more difficult to treat."

Add to the physical derailment the psychological manifestations that accompany Lyme, and you have children who are being told that their pains are all in their heads or who are suddenly labeled as learning disabled or victims of attention deficit disorder (ADD) and are funneled into neatly labeled classes and categories where they languish or continue their deterioration.

The best prevention is knowing what to look for and how to get help.

CHILDREN AND SYMPTOMS

The office of Dr. Charles Ray Jones (everyone tends to use his full name) mirrors the large print on his cream-colored walls, *The Land of Make Believe*. On the first floor of a professional building that sits on the apron of Yale University in New Haven, Connecticut, and near the student dormitories, this office is a child's playland, with a Little Tykes Kitchen, stuffed animals to calm the nerves, and videotapes, books, and pint-sized chairs all welcoming the smallest patients.

It is also a parents' wonderland in that the seventy-three-year-old pediatrician, who began professional life as a minister (Dr. Martin Luther King was a classmate), holds office hours seven days a week from 7 A.M. to 9 P.M., after which he takes and returns phone calls from all over the world, calming parents, consulting with foreign physicians, and handling emergencies. It is ironic that this large and gentle doctor, who has treated more than 4,000 of the smallest victims of Lyme disease with the philosophy "I treat until they're well," practices down the street from the institution that has bred and encouraged among both academics and insurance companies the dollar-saving philosophy that Lyme is cured in four weeks or less, despite any persistent symptoms, relapses, or patient deterioration. The recipient of the Lyme Disease Resource Center's Distinguished Physician Award, among many other community and professional honors, and a contributor to numerous studies regarding children and Lyme, Dr. Jones began treating Lyme patients "by default" more than thirty years ago when he first began noticing clusters of ill children with similar rheumatoid arthritic symptoms that cleared up with a course of antibiotics. Thousands of patients, years of research, and many "graduations" later—his office holds graduation ceremonies when a child gets well and is removed from antibiotics—he is so passionate about continuing the fight against the increasing number of tick-borne ailments he is seeing that he created an endowment three years ago at Columbia Presbyterian Hospital for a medical student interested in studying and treating Lyme and other tick-borne diseases.

The best advice he can give to parents, he says, is "trust your convictions. You know your child and you know when something isn't right. Don't give up. Contact Lyme disease support groups, go to your child's school and discuss what's happening with your child. Fewer than seven percent of my patients have had the bull's-eye rash, so don't rely on that. The problem isn't always Lyme, but Lyme has to be considered particularly in endemic areas."

His eyes, magnified behind thick lenses, grow sad when he talks of children who have died needlessly or have become permanently disabled. If only the treating doctors had believed the children's complaints, believed the parents, and, in some cases, particularly in hyperendemic communities, simply treated tick bites prophylactically with a benign course of antibiotics instead of taking a "wait and see what happens" attitude, he says, these tragedies would not have happened.

Most important, he says, is to pay attention to a child's complaints. "One child kept complaining that her 'hair hurt'—she was trying to describe pricks and a stabbing sensation in her scalp. Another child was scolded for dropping things, but he was having difficulty opening and closing his hands. Another child insisted on wearing dark glasses because his eyes were hypersensitive to light, and yet another began to go naked because his skin hurt."

Parents must educate themselves and remain vigilant. "If the mind doesn't know, the eyes don't see," says Dr. Jones.

The symptoms that children experience parallel those for adults, with emphasis on:

- Headache (more than 90 percent complain of this; they usually do not respond to over-the-counter analgesics)
- Sensitivity to light
- Dizziness
- Stiff neck
- Urinary frequency, burning, pain, or incontinence
- Bone or "hair" pain
- Eyes, blurry or loss of peripheral vision, eyelid twitches
- Hyperactive behavior
- Crying spells and depression
- Lost for words when speaking
- Backache
- Sleepiness
- Memory problems
- Difficulty concentrating
- Stomach pain (50 percent complain of this; a significant percentage may also have an ulcer)
- Mood swings and irritability (even in very young children)
- Chest pain (70 percent complained of this)
- Joint pain (primarily knees, wrists, and ankles)
- Sore throats ("The worse sore throat ever!" is a common complaint)
- Heart palpitations
- Tingling or numbness
- Rashes that come and go
- Letter and number reversals
- Pain caused by swelling of the optic nerve
- Bell's palsy

Children with central or peripheral nervous system involvement may also have wake-sleep disturbances, difficulty concentrating, episodes of disorientation, difficulty spelling words they could spell before the illness, and difficulty learning new material.

In attempting to describe symptoms, kids will be very specific—"my left knee" or "a headache at the front of my head." This type of complaint deserves attention.

Dr. Dorothy Pietrucha, a pediatric neurologist who practices on the New Jersey shore, says that children are susceptible to neurological infection from the spirochete. "I have seen children develop neurologic symptoms within a few weeks after a tick bite, while adults may not develop the symptoms for months or more. Many children are not diagnosed initially because their complaints are vague and are thought to be functional. One of the telltale situations is that the parents recall the child having a flu-like illness that preceded developing these rather persistent symptoms. Many claim that after this 'flu,' the child was never quite well or right again."

In a landmark study published in 1998 by Psychiatric Clinics of North America and led by Drs. Brian Fallon, Andrea Gaito, and Jennifer Nields, the underdiagnosis of neurologic Lyme in children was addressed for the first time. They found that in children and adolescents with neurologic Lyme disease, behavioral or mood disturbances are the second most frequently reported symptom, and that Lyme is capable of causing violent outbursts, panic attacks, and disorientation. Also, because of the onset of concentration difficulties, fatigue, headaches, and oppositional behavior, children and adults may ascribe new labels to children with Lyme. Children label themselves incompetent as they realize they can no longer keep up with their classmates, and teachers may label them as having ADD or as candidates for special education classes.

Among the study's conclusions is that while Lyme may be overdiagnosed in some rheumatology clinics, neurologic Lyme is being underdiagnosed, particularly where children are concerned.

It is easy to see from all this information that, though parents and teachers may be skeptical at first when presented with continual complaints, that in itself should be a red flag to pay attention.

THE "FAKING IT" MYTH

Despite such dismissal by some teachers and doctors, children do not fake Lyme disease or its symptoms. The reason is simple.

To do so would take too great a toll on the child, even if he or she could conceive and carry off such a plan.

"Kids ask why I've been so sick and I said, 'Lyme disease,'" said Billy. "They say, 'Lyme disease! Get away from me.' They think they can catch it and they won't play with me and they leave me out of things."

A major portion of a child's life is spent involved with school and friends. Yes, a child can fake one stomachache to get out of a math test. But children do not fake continually changing symptoms because the result may be the loss of social contact, being left behind in school, unpleasant medical treatment, and an inability to participate in previously enjoyed sports and activities.

No child would rather be declared chronically ill and have to do schoolwork at home, all by himself, for days on end. No child is going to give up Scouts, teams, field trips, overnights, parties, and music, dance, or riding lessons that are enjoyed. And no child can keep a charade going for the length of time the symptoms last in patients with Lyme.

"When Jenna said she couldn't use her arm and hand, my husband and I watched her at a friend's birthday party," said Ginny. "We thought maybe she'd forget and reach for something. But what we saw was a little girl trying desperately to enjoy the party and almost absentmindedly holding her numb arm with her good hand. That really convinced us."

Nobody knows a child like a parent does. Better than any doctor, teacher, or friend, a parent can tell when a child "isn't right," despite tests to the contrary. It is that inside knowledge regarding a child that places a parent in a position to be that child's advocate. And this is a very necessary position.

PARENTS AS ADVOCATES

When my son was first ill and we were going through the myriad tests to eliminate other problems, I quickly found that unless one spoke in a very insistent voice, it was easy to be relegated to a place in the woodwork. One lab did tests for our particular medical group, but tests were read only once a week because that was the group's day. Meanwhile, my child was getting worse on a daily basis.

It was absurd to wait a week for test results that were sitting on a desk, test results that would help determine the next step to my son's wellness. I expressed that feeling very clearly to the doctor and volunteered to pick up the tests and deliver them myself if he couldn't handle getting to the lab. We had the results read the following day and continued the process. My son could never have accomplished this on his own behalf. The complacency that sets in when routines are followed leads people to ignore desperate situations.

Growing up in a European-type household did not prepare me for having to fight authority figures, but when the realization dawned that the only thing standing between my child's life and possible death was me, I developed a different attitude. And *that* is what each of us must do for our children, whether we suspect they have Lyme disease or another difficult illness.

"You have to be an advocate for your child," agrees Carol Stolow, who with her husband, Bill, founded the Lyme Disease Network after her three daughters contracted Lyme. "Sometimes you have to take on the doctors, take on the school and teachers—everyone who's telling you what they think is wrong with your child. Sometimes they're looking for an easy 'out'; sometimes there's a different agenda. But your child needs to have representation in all of these arenas by someone who believes in and can fight for his or her rights."

Unfortunately, with Lyme, that advocacy is becoming important even in one's own household. Sometimes other family members doubt the diagnosis and question the child's motives in "acting sick." In a scattering of extreme cases, the controversy over a Lyme diagnosis and treatment is being used as a weapon in divorce cases, with one partner charging that the other is neurotically insisting a child is sick when he or she isn't and is therefore an unfit parent.

But nowhere does the child need an advocate more than at

school, where many teachers and administrators are still ignorant regarding the disease and its effects on children.

DEALING WITH SCHOOLS

Education is the best defense against Lyme disease, and one of the more important groups of people to educate is the educators—those individuals who see our children for a longer period of time than a parent does on any given school day. For it is in the classroom, and under stress, that Lyme symptoms will most commonly be apparent.

"I told the teacher I had a really bad headache at the front of my head," said eleven-year-old Tara. "She said, 'Oh, you have headaches every day. Can't you skip it today?'"

Nine-year-old Bill kept falling down during soccer practice. When he complained that his joints had been hurting and his ankles were weak, the coach scolded him for being a "weenie" and directed, "Play with pain. That's what the professionals do!"

Tina had been a strong A/B student all through her six years of school. Then, in seventh grade, her schoolwork began falling off, particularly math and Spanish. She complained of headaches and could barely stay awake in class. When she told her teachers that she was having trouble concentrating, they told her parents that Tina was becoming learning disabled and recommended both special-ed classes and a psychiatrist to help with her attention deficit disorder. Fortunately, Tina's doctor listened carefully and decided to test for Lyme disease. Tina's serology was positive, probably the result of a tick bite when visiting her cousins in California before school began.

For children, success in school is equated with success in life because school is, after all, their full-time job. When a child is infected with Lyme disease, physical symptoms impede the natural learning processes, and the child's credibility with the adults in charge becomes shaky. This further erodes the child's self-esteem for future performance.

Adding to the child's frustration and downward spiral are absences from school, resulting in pressure to catch up; isolation from or rejection by friends; and the frustration of attempting to learn when impaired memory and concentration, and other physical ailments, block learning receptors. It is important for educators to recognize a tick and know how to remove it, but it is not enough to merely stop there. Teachers and administrators need to be just as informed as physicians in recognizing the physical and psychological presentations of Lyme that they may see in the classroom.

This is a very real problem for many school districts, says John Staryak, supervisor of guidance services for the Jackson Township school district in New Jersey. At any given time, 15 to 20 percent of his student population can be down with Lyme disease. In most districts, when 30 percent of a school population has an illness, they close the schools.

"You can walk through the halls and look in classrooms, and you'll see kids with their heads down on the desks. These kids have Lyme disease, and it's become so common that the teachers and other kids in the class just accommodate it," says the tall, sandy-haired, former middle school teacher. "Unfortunately, this illness is impacting on the classroom, on the material, and on how teachers function in the class. I see us as having to deal with a whole different classification of learning-disabled student—they fall somewhere between chronically ill and learning impaired. And teachers need to have more in-services regarding the recognition of Lyme symptoms because we can't uniformly classify these students as perceptually impaired."

One school district that has created a proactive program of in-service training for teachers, school nurses, parents, and even children themselves is Greenwich Public Schools in Connecticut. When deputy superintendent Dr. Maria Melendez was confronted with the enormity of the problems that her district's families were facing, she brainstormed ways to educate the teachers to be more vigilant in recognizing the signs of Lyme in their pupils and to know how to deal with students who were fighting through the illness. With more than 9,000 students and 800 educators in fifteen buildings in one of the most Lyme-endemic areas of the country, this was no easy task.

Consulting with the Greenwich Lyme Discase Task Force, the health department, and her staff, Dr. Melendez decided to organize an informational evening seminar that would include a panel made up of some of the top doctors and advocates in the country. This videotaped evening has now been distributed across the nation to other school districts that request it, and is a compulsory part of new teachers' or nurses' school orientation in Greenwich.

"There is so much misinformation out there," says Dr. Melendez. "Change has to be a systemic effort. Just as we check for lice, checking children for ticks—particularly after sports or field trips—has to become part of the process until it becomes routine."

Among the other actions Melendez has spearheaded is the design of a protocol for students identified as being at risk for Lyme disease. This includes specific referral sheets that the adults in charge can use when a child has health complaints, as well as a school notification form for parents to fill out when they have a child with Lyme. The Greenwich school district also makes sure that the small tick removal kits designed by Time For Lyme are on all field trips and sports outings. In addition, because two of her fifteen schools are more than 40 percent Hispanic, Lyme disease information has been translated into Spanish as well.

"There has to be a partnership between the parents, the school, and the health department," says Melendez. "We need to recognize this and catch it early so we don't have children being funneled into special education classes who don't belong there. This is a disease that can be masked, and we want to do everything we can to avoid tagging children with a label they don't deserve."

Staryak agrees. "We have to look at students in a more individualistic and holistic way, with more attention paid to the pace of the individual than to the pace of the class.

"We need an alternative means of assessment for these students," says Staryak intently. "The easiest tests to correct are true-false tests, but this is where portfolio and contract learning come in. The Lyme disease student has difficulty storing and processing information. We need to teach students how to *manage* information, where to find and store it; in other words, the *process,* not the product, becomes the important thing. And that will be a very useful thing to teach all students."

The Individualized Education Program (IEP) is the cornerstone of the Individuals with Disabilities Education Act (IDEA) and ensures educational opportunities for all children suffering with a variety of disabilities, including Lyme disease. Required by law, it is an agreement to provide a specially designed educational program to meet your child's needs.

For Lyme patients, this may include at-home tutoring, a shorter school day, or supplemental instruction at the school. It is important to find out what is available in your particular school district that will assist your child in obtaining a good education.

If you think your child would benefit from an IEP, contact your local school board, your child's school, and your physician to get the appropriate forms and referrals. Then arrange to meet with your child's teachers and principal to discuss educational goals and the specific program. Do not let anyone bully you into thinking that they cannot accommodate you. It doesn't matter whether you live in a Lyme-endemic area or not. This is a federal law designed to serve the needs of families coping with a wide variety of illnesses and you are paying for this service through your taxes.

If the teachers in your child's school are unfamiliar with Lyme disease, you would be providing a major service by initiating a special information session through a local support group, hospital, public health agency, or informed doctor who is dealing with Lyme.

And finally, adjust your expectation level. We all have dreams for our children that often drive our plans, activities, and sacrifices. Suddenly, with Lyme disease, their healthy futures may be in jeopardy and our worlds are turned upside down. As one mother said, "It's normal to recognize the talents and abilities of your children and set goals and expectations that they will fulfill their potential. But with Lyme disease, normal goes out the window as do your dreams and expectations. What's left are your hopes and prayers that they simply will regain their health and live happy lives. That's it. That's really enough."

After all the pain, doubts, fears, and suffering children with Lyme have to go through, they need all the informed support possible in order to maintain a normal life. And those children in the adolescent-to-teenage range have an additional set of problems with which to cope.

9.
The Teenager

During the spring of his fifteenth year, my son Christopher was on his school's track and field team, learning to pole-vault, running three miles a day while listening to Air Force and Naval Academy motivational tapes, and actively participating in school projects. An honor student since elementary school, he was on the advanced track in both math and science in a rigorous northeastern private school. His easygoing manner and quick wit attracted numerous friends, and his plans for the next year included fulfilling a lifelong ambition—working toward his pilot's license, having already obtained his ham radio license the previous year.

During the summer, he went to the family pediatrician with several raised rashes on his legs and arms. The doctor diagnosed "summer rashes" and prescribed cortisone cream. A month later, Chris's glands were swollen, his throat sore, and his joints achy. The pediatrician treated him for mononucleosis and warned that it would take months to get over its effects.

That fall, Chris's grades began to slip. He grew alternately irritable and lethargic. He began to have trouble sleeping and felt dizzy and achy. He refrained from participating in school activities and stopped his trademark voracious reading. He broke up with his girlfriend and walked out on an aptitude test—something he normally found pleasantly challenging. When a school counselor suggested that Chris drop to a lower track in math and science, it was decided that all he needed was more discipline and less party time.

By Christmas, Chris was experiencing episodes of tremors, wherein his body would shake and twitch uncontrollably. The dizziness and pressure in his head were almost constant now. The pediatrician, after reviewing negative tests for brain tumors and MS, decided that Chris's cerebellum—the center of balance— was inflamed and prescribed Dramamine. Another month, four more doctors, and thousands of dollars in diagnostic tests later, the only suggestions from specialists were for Chris to see a psychiatrist for his increasing depression, irritability, lack of concentration, and episodes of tremors. School officials decided Chris must be on drugs. This "diagnosis" was proven false through a thorough drug screening.

Then, on Super Bowl Sunday, while at the home of good friends and in the midst of a congenial get-together, Chris had an episode of tremors that lasted two hours. By this time, I had read enough information on Lyme disease to demand the name of a Lyme specialist, despite several doctors' protests.

In the spring of his sixteenth year, Chris completed his second month of intravenous therapy, which had relieved most of his symptoms. After finishing the intravenous antibiotics, he was put on oral antibiotics following a relapse that brought back all of the original symptoms, including the tremors. He could not participate in sports; he had to drop chemistry, drop down a track in math, and anticipated repeating Spanish, because these three subjects depend on sequential learning—something of which he was incapable during the fall and winter. Despite the fact that he was dying to get his learner's permit to drive a car, he postponed that until he was confident that the tremors and dizziness were gone for good.

After ten months of antibiotics, he stopped taking them and, with a doctor's help, began to rehabilitate his body through nutrition, supplements, and exercise. Some days were very good and some days were bad.

On a bad day, he found it difficult to get up from the couch to answer the telephone, and depression was always a step away.

On a good day, he tended to overdo it in order to make up for all the days of feeling lousy—which usually backfired.

At the time of this writing, Chris is twenty-seven years old (hard for me to believe). He attended college, built an admirable reputation in the competitive IT world, and has a job that deals primarily with the pharmaceutical industry. He was reinfected once and treated swiftly with oral antibiotics. Over the last few years, he has experienced heart palpitations when under tremendous stress—something he attributes indirectly to Lyme.

"One thing about being sick for a long time—you know your body. You're more aware of how it works, how it reacts. As a teenager, you have medical words in your vocabulary that no one else knows—and you know what they mean. And sometimes you become overly aware of certain things going on in your body. When I was having chest pains, I went to a number of doctors, and after testing everyone said I was fine. One doctor finally said that when you are more aware of your body and heartbeat, you can become fixated on it and can literally send yourself into a panic attack. Part of the heart palpitations for me was a mental game. I realized it was always worse at night when I'd lie there feeling and thinking about the heartbeat. It's almost like having a flashback to a fear from the past.

"This last bout of flu, I started to think and worry that it's Lyme. It's always at the back of my mind, but I try not to be overly concerned. I know I am still in a high-risk group because I still hike, fish, and go out in the woods. If there's a tick I freak. I put on spray, cover up, and do tick checks afterward, but I know I'm exposing myself all the time. Then it goes back to the fact that I know my body and how it felt when I had Lyme. If I ever felt like that again, even the beginnings, I'd get to a doctor fast for antibiotics.

"It's important for teenagers to know that they *will* have a life again. It's hard to believe when you're going through the hell you go through with Lyme, but they will. And, like me, they will probably become better medical consumers because of it."

■ ■ ■

Although teens can usually articulate symptoms, there are so many other psychological and physiological processes going on during adolescence that doctors tend to look past the presenting symptoms for something more developmentally oriented— rebellion, raging hormones, drug abuse, and immaturity. Because of this, a significant percentage of teenage Lyme victims go undiagnosed until the condition is so severe that the child requires hospitalization, or until so many systems of the body are degenerating that serious attention is finally given.

Ask any adult if she or he would like to be fifteen again, and chances are the emphatic answer will be "No way!" Even at its best, adolescence is a pain for all concerned. There are issues of separation from parents, which touch off various forms of rebellion, the search for an identity and independence, and the exploration of new behaviors. There are social issues involving interaction with various hierarchies of society, including members of the opposite sex, and social choices regarding such things as alcohol, drugs, and sexual experimentation. And there are career goals and issues that propel the teen through a myriad of tests, options, and decisions.

Normal teens can experience mood swings, irritability, raging hormones that manifest in headaches, stress presenting as stomachaches, and a desire for individualization that is noticeable when they exhibit antisocial behavior around their parents.

Throw in a couple of curves like drug and alcohol experimentation, and is it any wonder that—without the benefit of seeing the rash (and not many parents see their teens' bodies unclothed)— parents, teachers, and doctors may have difficulty distinguishing where normal teenage angst ends and Lyme disease begins?

WHAT'S WRONG WITH THIS KID?

Fourteen-year-old Todd was found wandering the halls of the school. He received detentions for being "rebellious." The vice principal didn't believe him when, scared and upset, Todd told him he got lost.

Seventeen-year-old Wendy began falling down at school. Her lethargy, dropping grades, and inability to concentrate led the school counselor to recommend discipline for drug use.

Sixteen-year-old Jamie was becoming more and more frightened. Always a good student, his scores suddenly plunged in math, and he struggled in language arts. He realized that he was reversing numbers, in addition to having to deal with a constant headache and fatigue.

Unfortunately, in today's society, drug abuse is a legitimate concern when a teen's behavior and school performance change for the worse. This is probably the only age group where the first differential diagnosis that pops into mind is drug abuse, and so it must be ruled out before any credibility is given to any other diagnosis.

It doesn't make any sense to fight doing a drug screen. In fact, I would insist on it. The screen is a simple, noninvasive test. If it is positive, then you know you have one major problem to deal with; if it is negative, it just reaffirms that something else is wrong.

Apart from a drug screen, how can a parent, doctor, or educator distinguish between the normal teen problems and signs of Lyme?

"Look for chronicity," says Dr. Pietrucha. "This is where the patient history is most important. This is a child who is suddenly always sick. It is a teenager's nature to complain about a lot of things, but when you get right down to it, they go to school and get their work done.

"With Lyme, these kids become so unwell that they aren't capable of getting their work done, no matter what you say."

Drs. Fallon and Corsaro also recommend that you look for cognitive problems, including:

- Memory loss
- Disorientation

- Sudden onset of dyslexic tendencies
- Difficulty concentrating
- Sleep disturbances (insomnia; lethargy and sleepiness)

In addition, look for emotional instability such as overreactions and crying easily or suddenly. In reviewing dropped grades, pinpoint which subjects are plunging. If they are math, foreign languages, and science (such as chemistry), this is indicative of short-term memory and other cognitive problems.

Teens who are experimenting with drugs generally have a close circle of friends who are also involved. Teens who are infected with Lyme don't have the energy, stamina, or inclination to get together with friends.

Lyme presents the teen with frustrating problems that impinge on the normal issues of separation, identity, socialization, and goal setting. At a time when they are attempting to break away, they suddenly find themselves in a more dependent position because of their sickness and increasing psychological symptoms. At a time when they are trying to forge an identity, they are forced to defend their credibility if their symptoms are unbelieved, to the point of self-doubt and plummeting self-esteem. At a time when they should be learning new socialization patterns, the unpredictability of Lyme continually impedes their participation in social gatherings, commitments, and relationships. And at a time when they would normally be setting life and work goals, they are physically and emotionally restricted to fighting simply for wellness and perhaps watching certain dreams fade into the background.

Add to this the normal stresses of schoolwork and psychosocial development and you have a formula for a very unhappy camper.

If adults face ignorance about Lyme in the workplace and the medical field, teens don't fare much better. Despite the fact that they would normally rather have people think they hatched from eggs fully formed than admit they have parents who care, the teen Lyme patient, as well as the younger child, needs an advocate to represent him or her to those who unknowingly or uncaringly denigrate his or her rights and condition.

Then there are arrogant administrators such as the one who (though fully informed of fifteen-year-old Michael's condition and able to *see* he had an intravenous catheter in his arm) delivered the following "hit-and-run" message in the school hall before he strode on, leaving the struggling teenager devastated: "You know, I'm tired of you acting sick. You should be well by now!"

Or inconsiderate counselors like the one who commented to a seventeen-year-old Lyme patient, "Well, now that you're learning disabled, I guess you'll be looking into easy jobs instead of applying to college, huh?"

Or well-meaning overachieving fathers like the one who refused to let the school classify his daughter as chronically ill because he thought it would look bad on her college applications.

Like younger students, high school students are entitled to an Individualized Education Program (IEP) under federal law. With college looming on the horizon for many students, it is particularly important for you to be an advocate for your child and then, even after a program is created, it is up to you to make sure the school and the tutors live up to their commitment.

Leslie, whose two daughters both spent their high school years living with, and fighting Lyme disease, says that some of the tutors who were sent to the home were fabulous, but others would forget to show up. "You can never let up," she says. "You learn to be vigilant and basically have to stay in everyone's face to make sure your kids get the services they deserve."

College applications *are* a very real worry for many teens with Lyme, but hope and understanding are definitely at the end of the tunnel, as the effects of Lyme disease are being recognized by some of the country's major institutions.

THE COLLEGE APPLICATION DILEMMA

Since it is generally acknowledged that the junior year in high school is of utmost importance in the college application procedure, the worse-case scenario for a teen would then be to contract Lyme prior to the junior year and suffer through the year undiagnosed, or in the early stages of treatment.

Loss of time in school plus the cumulative physical and psychological effects of undiagnosed or chronic Lyme can add up to a year that is a washout in terms of grades and activities. And that's if the child is able to remain in school at all. There are many who have had to study at home on a long-term basis because they could not handle the day's unrelenting schedules.

Then too, there is the concern over taking the SATs—that standard yardstick used by most colleges in the admission process. Lyme disease certainly affects test-taking skills as much as it affects overall school performance. Because of the spread of Lyme disease, the Educational Testing Service, in Princeton, New Jersey, has made available an untimed SAT for which students can make application with supportive evidence from their doctors.

Lyme-literate physicians also become an integral part of their student-patients' college application procedures by writing letters of recommendation explaining the extenuating circumstances surrounding the students' records. These letters usually point out that the student was chronically ill during high school and for that reason grades may not have been up to what they would normally have been. They maintain that the student is presently improved and deserves the opportunity to study and get as complete an education as he or she desires.

"I've now had patients who have finished college and their grades and performance in college were considerably better than in high school," said Pietrucha. "They seem to be sickest during their high school years but then get on top of it. I'm optimistic that if a student gets treatment, even if he or she has some rough years, they can pursue a college education and further degrees if that's what they want."

College and tests aside, in the "black or white" world of teenagers, just getting through the disease is a major accomplishment. How do teens successfully cope? With a new awareness of their own mortality.

GETTING THROUGH IT—A NEW AWARENESS

Most of the kids Abby's age talk about rock stars, school tests, shopping malls, and the boys in class. Fourteen-year-old Abby's conversation is dotted with terms such as "spirochetes," "white-cell counts," "remitting and relapsing," and "encephalopathy." Her eyes fill with tears when she stops to think of how lonely she is, unable to join the other girls in normal social activities. Her Lyme went undiagnosed for more than two years. She is now into her tenth month of treatment, and her big goal in life is to be able to attend high school like a normal teenager.

"I feel like I am so far behind all the kids I used to hang out with," she says. "They are moving forward, making plans, *doing* things. I feel like a little kid, tied to medicines and my mommy. I don't want to live the rest of my life like this."

Chronic illness of any kind must be terribly frustrating. When it hits young people it carries a double whammy because the roller coaster of illness becomes a way of life.

Some doctors feel that teenage boys seem to cope better with Lyme disease by incorporating the necessary routines into their schedules and displaying a more optimistic attitude regarding wellness than some girls, who have tried to take overdoses of sleeping pills to end the pain. On occasion, the frustration over the needless intensity of the illness due to lack of knowledge and diagnosis of Lyme overtakes some teens, who exhibit a rage response. These are usually isolated instances, however. If this type of reaction becomes part of the everday pattern, then it would be wise to seek counseling for that child.

Actually, for those who are in the chronic stage of Lyme, counseling can provide many benefits, if only to help the teen deal with a long-term illness and assure him or her that he or she is not going crazy.

Connor was bitten by a tick when he was three and was finally diagnosed with Lyme when he was six. Today, he is six-teen years old and the last time he spent a full school day in a classroom he was seven years old. During the intervening years, he lost his hearing twice, suffered seizures, pain all over his body, and other aspects of neurologic Lyme. He also testified before Congress on the need for funding for Lyme disease research. His family moved from endemic New Jersey to the coast of North Carolina three years ago and he made a conscious decision to leave as much of his Lyme history behind as possible, since he found that the kids treated him as if he *were* the disease. Today, he is optimistic about the future and has a few words of advice for other teenagers going through it.

"When I first got Lyme, it was like I had gotten run over by a car. Many people know what I'm talking about when I say I couldn't remember things that had happened to me just five minutes beforehand. I also couldn't get out of bed because I was so tired and fatigued. My joints started acting up, I would have all sorts of aches and pains, and the part that I hated most was that some people didn't even believe me! Many people would see me in class, and because I couldn't focus on the task at hand, they would think that I was making up my sicknesses because I wanted to get out of my work.

"However, all of those ailments were nothing compared to when I started having seizures and vertigo. They were, and still are, by far the worst things that I had ever felt in my life. It was like I had never experienced any type of feeling or emotion before. After feeling those, and finding out about what was causing them, I thought that I would never feel well again. I kept that frame of mind until I met doctors like Dr. Dorothy Pietrucha, who knew and treated kids with cases like mine. After treating me, Dr. Pietrucha helped me to feel better and enjoy life. I would not have made it this far in my life, were it not for Dr. Pietrucha. I owe more than I can give to her. Many other people I'd like to thank include Dr. Robert Bransfield, Dr. Kenneth Liegner, Dr. Richard Neubauer, Dr. Brian Fallon for speaking several times at my school, Leslie Salmon for her guidance, all of my tutors over the years, and Denise Lang for letting me say all of this.

"One thing that I must impart upon all who read this,

whether you have this disease or someone you know has it, is that the downs of this disease are not permanent. With the right doctors and enough time a person with Lyme can, and will, get better. I also would like to give some hints, though these are not for everyone. They're my little, nonmedical cures for when I have certain symptoms.

"Whenever I'm tired or fatigued, I drink black pekoe tea, though I have learned to drink different types of tea for different symptoms. I only drink coffee if I need a quick boost, though it is up to you whether you want to drink tea or coffee.

"Whenever I'm depressed, I listen to music or watch comedy shows. I've found that comedy can cheer a person up in any type of mood. If ever I need to escape the troubles of my world, I read or write. I read because I imagine myself to be the character, so I can forget my problems. I write because writing is a great form of self-expression, along with things like painting and songwriting. Unfortunately, there aren't many more ways to fix a symptom of Lyme, nonmedically. But I wish the people who have Lyme or know someone who has it good luck."

Like Connor, teens themselves find various methods of getting through the tedium of feeling unwell, stymied activities, and academic struggles.

"Don't doubt yourself," says Kelly, sixteen. "And try not to let doctors bully you into doubting yourself. Remember, there are still a few good doctors who will try their best to find a cure for you."

Seventeen-year-old Chris, my son, recommends that teens focus on short-term goals. "Find something to look forward to—a concert, a party, getting together with a friend you haven't seen in a long time—something that you can set your mind on when your body is feeling lousy. Also, it helps to have an outlet for those feelings of frustration. I took up the drums and it really helps; it's also good exercise and I feel better after I've played."

"Try to keep to as normal a routine as possible," says Jeremy, fifteen. "I know some kids with Lyme find it hard to even get out of bed, but it's important to try to do all the regular things. I like to take a walk around the block and look at the people and things around me."

All the teens I spoke to agree that keeping in touch with friends is very important, even during those times that they felt the worst. It helped to focus their attention on something outside themselves and their aches and pains.

One word of caution, however. With chronic or late-stage Lyme there are so many days when the teen feels crummy that on those few days when the symptoms blend into the background, the child wants to pour all of his or her energy into activities in a seemingly frantic attempt to make up for lost time. This can lead to overexertion, which inevitably results in a physical and emotional "crash" afterward. It is difficult for a parent to apply the "brakes," so to speak, particularly when you empathize with your child's desire to be "normal," but it is advisable.

Finally, teenagers with Lyme need support not only from their parents but from other teens who are fighting the same fight they are. Contact your local Lyme support group and ask the leader if the group includes teenagers. If not, check with other schools to see if they have any students who are down with Lyme and hook your teenager up with them. When my son was in high school, he made up flyers and sent them to every school in the area to say that he would be available to talk with other kids who had Lyme and needed to connect. He took many calls and I honestly think he got at least as much out of helping and sharing his ordeal as the teenagers who called him for advice and an empathetic ear.

Although Chris had specific hours posted for call-ins, I'll never forget the call that came just before he got home from school. It was from a young girl, who asked in a trembling voice, "I'm not going to die from this, am I? I don't want to ask my parents because they're too worried. But so am I."

One by-product of teenage Lyme is that the youngsters involved develop an awareness of their own mortality that is not common in most kids their age.

"I think I'm more careful when I drive, and I tend to look out for the other kids I'm with," says Jean, seventeen and a Lyme patient for two years. "Sometimes I feel more like their mother than their friend, but I know I can die. I don't think I'm immortal. I came too close to dying or at least feeling like I was going to die, with Lyme. Maybe, after I'm cured, I'll forget these feelings, but for right now, I try to appreciate the good moments."

10.

Women

During the summer of 1994, thirty-five-year-old Derya went on a golf outing that changed her life.

For this AT&T manager, a vivacious dynamo who rides a Harley-Davidson on weekends, the day of golfing was one of the many perks of achieving outstanding sales and performance for the communications giant located in the lush, rolling hills of northern New Jersey. Derya spent a great day on the course, but by evening her right elbow was in pain.

Over the course of the next couple of weeks, the pain moved into her wrist, arm, and shoulder and across her shoulders into her left arm and fingers. She just attributed it to her active lifestyle, until an overpowering weakness invaded her arms and hands and she found it difficult to hold on to the steering wheel of her car.

By the end of September, she was diagnosed with lupus. When her blood tests came back negative she went to an internist. She was now experiencing pain in her neck, cheeks, and lips, and muscle spasms in her thighs and eyes. When she got her period, her symptoms got worse.

Both at work and home, Derya became frightened as she struggled with memory loss, fatigue, and headaches. "And I would open my mouth to speak, and something completely different than what I intended would come out!" she says. "You can't do business like that!"

Over the course of the next couple of months, her skin, now very sensitive, began to hurt so badly that she couldn't bear to be touched. "This did not do wonders for my marriage," she says. "And I was irritable all the time."

She saw infectious-disease doctors, allergists (for bouts of sneezing and a left-side sort throat), and a husband-wife medical team who diagnosed her with AIDS.

"You know, when I had the female doctor, I thought at least I'd be taken seriously. Some of the other doctors would listen to me as I listed all of my complaints and think I was an hysterical female looking for attention." Then when she mentioned the fact that all the symptoms seemed worse during her period, the doctors became patronizing and wrote off the complaints as a severe case of PMS.

Although one of the doctors along the way had tested her for Lyme disease with a Western Blot, apparently he didn't know how to read the results, since five of the bands came out positive.

After hearing the AIDS diagnosis, Derya became hysterical. The doctor then hedged and said, "Well, it *could* be MS." So she underwent another round of tests. Despite the positive Western Blot, the doctor refused to treat her with antibiotics because "it would make all the other tests come out negative."

By this time, unable to work consistently, and completely fatigued at home, Derya had to go on disability. She found that all she could do was lie in bed. She didn't trust doctors anymore and didn't want to be touched because she was in such pain. All she wanted to do, she said, was die.

Finally, a concerned family member convinced her to call 888-366-6611, a hot line sponsored by the Lyme Disease Association, which gave her the names of five doctors in the same general geographic region who could treat her properly.

Derya finally got the treatment she needed, and went on a program of antibiotics, nutrition, and adjunctive chiropractic care. Today, Derya suffers from chronic Lyme but is in the hands of a lyme-literate physician. She knows when she's beginning to have a relapse because of the "jackhammer headache and the whoosh that you feel when you go to move your head—it's a headache like no other you've ever felt in your life. And around the time of my period, it's the worst!" Her dark eyes still flash in anger when she recalls her medical maze and the way she was treated by physicians along the way.

"Because you are a woman, you're told you're menopausal, you're crazy and need psychological counseling, you're hysterical, you need a better sex life—anything not to take you seriously," she says.

All too many women have found that they are not given credibility by medical personnel, both when they are the patients and when they are the advocates for their children.

"It really burns me," agrees Leslie Salmon, who has had to fight for her daughters' Lyme treatment in the face of medical ignorance, insurance company nonpayments, and hassles from the girls' school system. "Why is it that you can document everything, discuss symptoms with the doctor, give a time line, reactions to medications—everything to do with the child you know so well in a perfectly calm voice, and all you have to do is have your husband with you for a visit and, right away, the doctor defers to the male, who for the most part knows much less than the mother in the house?"

YOU DON'T LOOK SICK

Another form of discrimination against women who are attempting to seek a medical diagnosis of Lyme comes in the form of presentation. That is, most women tend to be concerned with their appearance no matter where they go or how rotten they feel. This is especially true of Lyme patients who "don't look sick" in the first place, despite their bodies and minds falling apart on the inside. More than a few women have been told by physicians, "Well, you say all of these things are wrong with you but you look too good to be that sick!"

Should women dress down, leave off the makeup, and arrive at the doctor's office with hair that hasn't been washed for days?

Make your own decision, but know that you aren't alone in experiencing this discrimination.

LYME-RELATED YEAST INFECTIONS

Once a woman is on a course of antibiotics for her Lyme disease, another medical complication can arise that women frequently don't associate with Lyme. Extended treatment with strong antibiotics can reduce the flora in the intestinal lining that stave off bad bacteria. The result can be a massive yeast infection (for more on candida, see chapter 18). Although millions of women have experienced vaginal yeast infections during their lives for a variety of reasons, few are prepared for the severity of symptoms resulting from antibiotic treatments for Lyme, including blisters in the soft tissues of the extremely swollen genitals. Women should be aware of these manifestations and see a doctor immediately, should they develop.

"I was horrified," said one woman. "I thought my husband might have been having an affair and brought some sexually transmitted disease home. And he was thinking the same thing about me! Why don't doctors warn us about these things?"

A STUDY OF WOMEN AND LYME

Because of some of the unique problems affecting women with Lyme disease, special research is being conducted that should add legitimacy to female complaints during the illness.

Dr. Mary Lynn Barkley, a neurobiologist with the University of California at Davis, launched a study in conjunction with Dr. Nick Harris of IgeneX that examined the effects of menstrual hormonal changes on the spirochete and the resulting symptoms. Through clinical trials she's found that, regardless of antibiotic therapy, Lyme disease symptoms are exacerbated every twenty-eight days when a woman's hormonal production shifts, thus influencing immune system function.

We found that there is definitely a flare in symptoms in women who have regularly recurring menses," says Barkley. "There is also an indication that there's a window of time at the end of the menstrual cycle that coincides with an increased ability to detect Lyme in the woman's urine."

Harris says that this will benefit women who had been clinically treated for persistent Lyme disease but had never had a positive laboratory marker for the disease. Urine samples collected at the start of menses for three to five days were positive for Lyme antigen, thus supporting the clinical diagnosis of Lyme disease. For this reason, IGeneX has been refining a more sensitive Lyme urine antigen test that will assist in future diagnoses.

Barkley says that the study regarding women and more intense symptoms during menses confirms what doctors and patients have been reporting for years. She is currently working with a research group in Italy on the study of hormones—specifically how the drop in progesterone levels during menses affects women's immune systems and leaves them more vulnerable to things like Lyme disease.

It is bad enough when adults and children contract Lyme disease and it goes undiagnosed. However, it is especially frustrating and guilt-inspiring when an infected mother is not recognized as having Lyme and passes that disease to her unborn child.

11.
The Pregnant Woman

It is estimated that 20 percent of the patients with Lyme disease in both North America and Europe are women between the ages of 20 and 49; in other words, women in their prime childbearing years.

When a pregnant woman contracts Lyme disease, not only does she run the risk of progressively debilitating symptoms that parallel progressive infection, so does her unborn baby. Medical documentation indicates that there is a transfer of the spirochetes from the mother's body through the placenta to the fetus.

A study by Dr. Jack Remington of Stanford University and Dr. Jerome Klein of Boston University showed that this in utero infection by the Lyme organism can result in stillbirth, spontaneous abortion, and damage to the brain, heart, liver, and other organs. Or it can result in the newborn's living a life of chronic illness that baffles pediatricians, puts stress on the family, and prevents the child from growing, thriving, and socializing within the normal parameters of development.

A FAMILY ILLNESS

Lynn had everything going for her when she was bitten by an infected tick on vacation during the summer prior to her wedding. She held a high-powered job as a financial analyst in New York City, she was engaged to be married, and her outgoing nature kept her in a whirl of outdoor and social activities. By her September wedding date, two months later, she had been treated for a virulent "flu," had been diagnosed as having shoulder problems, and underwent an appendectomy. Four months later, another doctor said she had thyroid problems, depression, and menstrual irregularities. By September of the following year, she was so chronically ill that she had to give up her job.

Not only did this put a strain on her new marriage, but during her pregnancy a year later she experienced increasingly varied symptoms, culminating in a neurologic stroke. At least baby Lauren was healthy, she thought desperately, when she was told in the delivery room that the Apgar score was perfect.

That jubilation lasted only four months, however, because the infant soon developed ring rashes all over her ankles. At five months, she began experiencing a series of chronic ear infections, and by seventeen months she suffered from severe pneumonia. Repeated trips to pediatricians and specialists could not uncover the causes of the continual stomach pains, sore throats, recurring fevers, and chronic illness.

Although Lynn herself was continually sick, she tried to keep a low profile on her own aches and pains as she tended her sick child and nursed the hope that the new child she was carrying would be born in good health. But this second pregnancy only exacerbated her varied symptoms and led her to be hospitalized at New York City's Columbia Presbyterian Hospital for a repeated series of tests that kept proving negative.

Jack was born five weeks premature and seemed to be ill from the beginning. He cried fourteen hours a day, gained very little weight, suffered from the same upper respiratory problems as his sister, and screamed when he urinated.

As Lynn saw both her children struggle to survive, and a plethora of doctors pass them around, a rage built inside that motivated her to begin taking medical courses at the local university. But the knowledge that the courses brought could not stop her own deterioration, which led to surgery for damage to her liver and pancreas. For the next two years, she made the rounds of doctors who were looking for autoimmune disorders, doctors who inspired her to examine her life for illness-oriented behaviors, and doctors who told her that her problems and those of her children were all in her head.

Then after she and her children suffered agonizing bouts of "flu," chicken pox, and heart problems, Lynn tested positive for Lyme disease. Shortly, thereafter, her children were diagnosed with congenital Lyme. All began treatment.

Today, Lauren has an abnormal EEG that indicates temporal lobe seizure disorder, an abnormal MRI, and hyperactivity disorders. Jack suffers from sensory deficiencies, migrating pain, and attention deficit disorder aggravated by the Lyme.

"We have to prevent the late diagnosis of Lyme and make sure that all pregnant women who suspect they have Lyme disease get to knowledgeable doctors who will treat them aggressively to prevent what happened to my children," says Lynn.

"I keep telling myself that we'll beat this thing," she says, her eyes filling. "I made a promise to myself. I have to do this for my son, who wakes up in the middle of the night and cries to please make the pain go away. I have to do this for my daughter, whose fists I have to hold as she's crying and trying to hit me in a confused and painful rage. And also for my father, who at age fifty-seven has been told he has permanent brain damage now because of Lyme and that if it had been diagnosed five years ago, he wouldn't have this.

"People have to hear the true story of what Lyme disease can do to your life and the lives of those you love."

The studies done on pregnancy and Lyme disease are still too few. According to Dr. Louis Bracero, associate professor of obstetrics and gynecology at New York Medical College, Lyme disease follows the pattern of other spirochetal illnesses that are contracted via the placenta during pregnancy. Lyme spirochetes have been found in the liver, heart, and other organs of babies who were born to women with Lyme and who died. A study by Dr. Alan MacDonald, of Southampton Hospital in New York, revealed that Lyme disease acquired in utero may result in fetal death either in utero or shortly after birth. He also discovered that tissue inflammation was not seen in fetuses that acquired Lyme disease through the placenta, and that in all but one of the cases where the Lyme organism was identified in the placenta or the fetal tissues, the maternal blood had no evidence of antibodies to the Lyme bacteria.

Continuing research regarding transplacental Lyme is being undertaken by the Lyme Disease Foundation in Tolland, Connecticut, which examines placentas for evidence of spirochetes, but many more studies are needed.

There is a concern among pregnant women who have tested positive for Lyme in the past, successfully completed treatment, and remain asymptomatic that their babies still might acquire Lyme in utero. Some have even expressed confusion over whether their pregnancies should be terminated.

Drs. Len Sigal and Ana Fernandez, of the Lyme Disease Center, Robert Wood Johnson Medical School, feel that while pregnancy complicated by Lyme disease should not be terminated, treatment of the mother's Lyme should be undertaken immediately to prevent ensuing complications. This view is also held by experts across the country and is included in *Conn's Current Therapy*, the treatment "bible" of physicians, which says that the likelihood the fetus will be infected through the placenta is highest early in the disease, when it is being quickly disseminated by the blood. For this reason, a pregnant woman who contracts Lyme, particularly during the first trimester of pregnancy, should be treated aggressively with antibiotics. There is a risk throughout the entire pregnancy, however, that the mother will pass the spirochetal infection to her unborn infant, and experts also advise that treatment would seem to be indicated throughout the pregnancy for the best protection for the baby.

While this would seem to be fairly straightforward advice regarding pregnancy and Lyme, the obstacle once again is diagnosis, and pregnant women face nearly as much prejudice as do teenagers.

"OH, YOU'RE JUST PREGNANT!"

Being a mother is everything to Diane, who lives in Pennsylvania. "My kids are my life," cheerfully states this mother of four with another on the way. This, her fifth pregnancy, has brought about a whole set of problems and prejudices, however, that Diane never expected to encounter.

She doesn't remember a tick bite, but she distinctly remembers the beginning of her symptoms early in her pregnancy. First came the stiff neck, swollen glands, lump in her throat, headaches, and incredible fatigue. By the end of June (two months into the pregnancy), she had pain in her chest when she took a breath. When she told her obstetrician, he said, "You're pregnant. Pregnant women are supposed to get aches and pains." After the chest pains, he blamed her aches on a lack of sleep and prescribed Tylenol with codeine. Despite the fact she protested that she knew what the aches of pregnancy were and this was different, that she didn't feel "right," she was told it was because of her condition.

A month later, while on vacation, she had to be rushed to a hospital emergency room with what she thought was a heart attack. Tests revealed nothing. Maybe it was bronchitis, the doctors suggested.

Ensuing symptoms included chills (during warm weather), continued chest pain, blurred vision, light-headedness, and hypersensitivity of her legs, back, and head. Diane tried to explain this to her doctor again—and to a couple of specialists along the way. She was told, "Go home and do Lamaze breathing and everything will be fine."

By this time she had heard of Lyme disease, and she requested information on it. "Oh, it's the 'in' disease to have right now. Don't worry about it," said the doctor.

She thought her problems were over when she was finally put in touch with a doctor who did see Lyme cases, but she was told that despite the fact that he suspected Lyme, he wouldn't treat pregnant women. Seeking help from the University of Pennsylvania, she was told that they would treat her only if she would transfer all of her records to them and have her baby there. Though she felt she couldn't do that, they gave her two weeks' worth of antibiotics, which she took.

"For five days I felt normal," she says. "Then I got a burning in my joints and the pain in my head came back. I went to a rheumatologist, who would not even test me for Lyme because he said that if I had been on antibiotics for two weeks I was cured.

"At seven months pregnant, I'm still not feeling good. I get strange headaches, feel out of it. The pain has been so horrible that I've even packed my head in ice to try and stop it. Nothing works, and no one will treat me. They say to come back after I give birth if I still have a problem. I went to a neurologist who told me I'd feel better after the baby was born. I was worried about the baby so I went to a perinatalogist, who checked and said the baby looks okay but is several weeks behind in developing.

"I'm very worried, with all the evidence of stillbirths and miscarriages. Every doctor has blamed my pregnancy and the fact that it is my fifth child," says Diane heatedly. "I got so tired of hearing it, I wanted to punch them! Believe me, I'm happy to be pregnant—I wanted this—but what I'm feeling isn't pregnancy. It's different, and when I feel the pains, I have to wonder, 'What do I do now?'"

A growing number of ob-gyns, particularly those in Lyme-endemic areas of California, Wisconsin, Connecticut, New York, and New Jersey, are treating patients prophylactically during the first trimester of pregnancy if they are bitten by ticks or present Lyme symptoms. Dr. Peter Bippart, who is a member of an ob-gyn group in Morristown, New Jersey, sees a significant number of women who have Lyme disease, or are in real danger of contracting it due to tick bites that they have reported.

"In our practice, we will treat a patient with amoxicillin for about three weeks, especially during the first trimester. It is just not worth the risk to ignore it," says Dr. Bippart. "Especially when you consider that the antibiotic treatment is so benign."

MY LITTLE MIRACLE

Laura Mucci, twenty-seven, has suffered with Lyme since she was diagnosed at age thirteen. Growing up in Lyme-endemic New Jersey, she spent her high school years in pain, shuttling between doctors' offices. She fought to graduate with her class and, in a wheelchair part-time, attended college. Her parents were thrilled three years ago when she married a man who had cheered her along all through her illness. Finally, her parents thought, she would begin a normal life. Still battling chronic Lyme, even while Laura was working and attending graduate school, her spirit seemed indomitable. But when she announced that she was pregnant with the family's first grandchild, her mother panicked.

"I was terrified for her and terrified for her unborn child," says her mother, Leslie, whose other two children also suffer from chronic Lyme disease. "For so many years, I wondered if there would be life after Lyme disease. While I was excited by the thought of a grandchild and could see how happy Laura was, deep down inside I was so scared. I've seen what Lyme can do."

Laura, too, was afraid—but more afraid that she would be responsible for bringing a child into the world who would be chronically ill. She immediately consulted the physician who had guided her to wellness so many times, Dr. Joseph Burrascano. "He was so happy for me," she says. "But he immediately put me on antibiotics—pregnant women can only take amoxicillin and Ceftin safely—and then referred me to a high-risk pregnancy physician, Dr. Judy Banks, closer to home who monitored me carefully. I stayed on antibiotics throughout my pregnancy and everything went wonderfully well."

Today, baby Michael is the picture of health at two years old—something Laura doesn't take for granted. "Because of Lyme, I only remember half of my childhood. I remember fifteen spinal taps. I remember headaches that wouldn't stop. But if this is my reward for all that pain, it was worth it. Michael is my miracle and I've never been happier. We are thinking about having a second child and when I told Dr. Burrascano, he laughed and said,

'Go for it.' But then I wonder if I'm pushing my luck because Michael is so perfect. I always think of Lyme; it's always with me. I still have good and bad days, but you have to go on with your life. You just have to be smart about it.'"

SEEKING HELP AND COPING

Although informed medical viewpoints are slowly spreading, the norm is unfortunately more like the treatment given Diane, particularly in those areas where a massive denial of Lyme disease is prevalent.

If you are pregnant and have been bitten by a tick in an endemic area, are displaying symptoms consistent with Lyme disease, or have been diagnosed with Lyme in the past:

1. Don't accept ignorance or denial from your doctor. During pregnancy, time is of the essence in getting antibiotic treatment to protect your baby if you have, or have been exposed to, Lyme disease. It is important to treat tick bites in endemic areas prophylactically; the comparative risk is minimal.

2. If your doctor refuses to consider Lyme disease, seek help from your local Lyme support group (see appendix B) to locate a high-risk pregnancy obstetric specialist. Whether the test is positive or negative is irrelevant. If the clinical diagnosis can be made, it is recommended that you be treated right through delivery and beyond. Your ob-gyn should remain in close communication with your treating physician. The risks to both you and your unborn child by not treating Lyme with antibiotics are simply not worth taking.

3. Don't doubt yourself. If this is a first pregnancy, you may be unaware of the aches and pains that pregnancy causes. If, however, you are not improving or if your symptoms are "different" from those of previous pregnancies and it is possible that you were exposed to Lyme, don't feel "dumb" going back to your doctor and reporting your symptoms.

4. After the birth, be vigilant in your observations regarding the health of your baby. Even though a baby born to a Lyme mother may

appear to be healthy at the moment of birth, it is still possible that transplacental Lyme symptoms can crop up months later. There is no need to be paranoid and neurotic about this; just be observant and consider the possibility if chronic illness becomes a way of life for your infant.

5. Breast-feeding is also not recommended if you have had Lyme disease during the previous year, since Lyme spirochetes have been isolated from breast milk.

A pregnant woman worries about a lot of things that will affect her baby's health—and rightly so. It is important that doctors realize that, far from being hysterical, most women today are somewhat knowledgeable about their bodies and various health and environmental threats. Complaints of diffuse and migratory symptoms during pregnancy should be treated with respect, not simply dismissed as "pregnant women's blues," curable through Lamaze breathing. Pregnant women must expect and demand this respect and treatment—and seek additional help when they don't receive them.

Pregnant women and teens are not the only groups of people who face prejudice or special circumstances surrounding the diagnosis and treatment of Lyme. Senior citizens—however that age is defined—also find that they are lumped into a group with an expected pattern of illness or behavior.

12.

The Elders

Consider this: according to the Alzheimer's Disease Association, the following ten symptoms are warning signs of Alzheimer's:

- Recent memory loss that affects job performance
- Difficulty performing familiar tasks
- Problems with language
- Disorientation of time and place
- Poor or decreased judgment
- Problems with abstract thinking
- Misplacing things
- Changes in mood or behavior
- Changes in personality
- Loss of initiative

Sound familiar? As if that isn't scary enough, the National Institute on Aging warns that the term *dementia* describes a group of symptoms that are caused by changes in brain function. Dementia symptoms include asking the same questions repeatedly, becoming lost in familiar places, being unable to follow directions, and getting disoriented about time, people, and places.

These warnings are coupled with the fact that 76 million baby boomers are heading into what are considered "senior" years. The Society of Actuaries recently released predictions that "if science can't combat the disabilities of old age, suicide (predicted to account for 13 out of every 100,000 deaths in the next five years) may seem the only alternative."

If children and women face overriding prejudices and lack of credibility among health care professionals, it is frighteningly worse for the elderly who, when they begin to complain of muscle aches, dizziness, and an inability to concentrate or remember, are dismissed with "Well, this is to be expected as you're getting older." Considering that the two most afflicted age groups for Lyme disease are those under ten and over fifty, this could add up to a crisis situation within the next five years.

When sixty-four-year-old Tony returned home from a driving vacation through Florida with his wife, he began falling apart. First, he began to forget things—where he was going, what he was doing, the names of friends and relatives. His joints ached so badly that he lost the ability to walk and even to feed himself. Dizzy and confused, he retreated from speaking with people.

When medical help was sought, Tony was quickly diagnosed as having Alzheimer's disease. Three months after he returned from his active trip to Florida, Tony was admitted to a nursing home, incontinent, disoriented, and strapped to a chair to prevent him from falling out.

His distressed daughter, remembering something she had read about Lyme disease, contacted Dr. Derrick DeSilva and asked for an evaluation. After taking a thorough history from family members, reviewing Tony's medical deterioration, and performing an examination and ordering supportive tests, a diagnosis of Lyme disease was made. Tony was put on intravenous antibiotics.

Six weeks later, Tony was once again able to move under his own power, control his bodily functions, and return to his normal life at home, while continuing antibiotic treatment.

A case like Tony's dramatically demonstrates how a "catch-all" diagnosis like Alzheimer's can misdirect a doctor's attention from important diagnostic issues when dealing with the older

patient. Older citizens get aches and pains; they sometimes suffer a form of dementia. In the not-too-distant past, "Oh, he's
just senile" would cover all the bases, including those that caused
a personality change as well. It was easy to write off senior citizens because, after all, they were expected to be sickly and
would probably die soon anyway.

Today, when modern medicine has allowed us to live longer
and octogenarians are the fastest-growing age group, even the
term "elderly" or "senior citizen" causes confusion. Does one
recognize a fifty-year-old as a senior citizen, as does the American Association of Retired Persons (AARP)? Or do we address
the sixty-five-year-old, who is finally eligible for Medicare, as
"senior citizen"? At what point do doctors expect people to
begin falling apart?

Ask any of the baby boomers—who cut their teeth on shat-
tering established institutions during the 1960s and '70s, and
now spend their forties, fifties, and even sixties starting new
careers, creating businesses, and redesigning their bodies to
accommodate a longer, ideally healthier life span—and you'll see
that the formerly accepted notion of aging and disability has
fallen by the wayside. So why are medical professionals so quick
to ascribe Alzheimer's—a legitimate and truly terrible disease—
to anyone over sixty who seems to be failing?

A CHALLENGING DIAGNOSIS

With Lyme disease, these issues can be very real obstacles to
diagnosis. So can the fact that, frequently, older citizens with
Lyme may have symptoms masked by other ills such as diabetes,
arthritis, ALS, hypertension, heart problems, and some mild form
of dementia. Add to that a prevailing prejudice against the credibility of an older person's memory, and once again we have a
situation where a patient must fight to be believed prior to even
establishing the illness—and another situation in which an aggressive and caring advocate becomes the patient's best tool for getting proper medical care.

Janice's mother, an active and alert seventy-seven-year-old, began having bouts of falling down. Her heart would race; her personality began to change. Knowing that her mother was an avid gardener who lived in a Lyme-endemic area of Maryland, Janice contacted her doctors and requested that they give her mother an ELISA and Western Blot in addition to their EEGs and other battery of tests. The doctors refused because the request had to come from their patient, not the patient's long-distance daughter, and Janice's mother—being from a generation that didn't question a doctor—didn't want to "upset him" by making requests. After getting the negative results from tests targeting everything from heart disease and diabetes to lupus and ALS, Janice was told that her mother "most likely had Alzheimer's" and they should both get used to the idea that she would need to get a wheelchair.

This time, Janice traveled to Maryland and, in her mother's presence with the doctor, requested the ELISA and Western Blot. This time the doctor, with a dismissive attitude, agreed. Over the course of the next two weeks, Janice had to make seventeen telephone calls to the doctor's office in order to get test results, as she watched her mother continue to deteriorate. She finally drove to the doctor's office and confronted him. "Oh yes," he said, "the results are right here. The ELISA was negative, but the Western Blot looks faintly positive, if you want to put your faith in that."

"I think he gave my mom a course of antibiotics just to shut me up, but when she began to show marked improvement, he started to pay attention," says Janice. Today, her mom is back to gardening, attending her book club, and taking monthly day trips with her senior church group. "My mother would have never fought for a test and results like I did. She was ill and really more concerned that the doctor would think she was just another old pain in the behind."

Having made it into their seventies and eighties, some older citizens do have a lot of health baggage and may already be on several other medications. This has an impact on a diagnosis of

Lyme because other antibiotics may cause a false negative test, and other illnesses can cross-react to cause a false positive. For these reasons, the clinical diagnosis leans heavily, once again, on the patient's history.

History taking is the most important tool a doctor can use at any time, but even more so with an older patient. But since they may not be able to give it themselves, it is the doctor's responsibility to talk at least to the children to get an accurate work, vacation, and leisure time history. There needs to be an evaluation as to whether the symptoms are part of an acute illness or chronic illness, and if the patient is suffering from delirium, whether this is acute as well.

Those patients who are in nursing homes with diagnoses of dementia should be tested for Lyme disease. There is a difference between acute delirium brought about because of Lyme and degenerating dementia caused by other illnesses. The type of dementia caused by Lyme is reversible if it is caught and treated early on in the disease.

Studies in recent years, performed in sites ranging from Rush-Presbyterian-St. Luke's Medical Center in Chicago to North Shore University Hospital in Manhasset, Long Island, concern the possible connection between the Lyme spirochete and diseases normally associated with the aged, such as Alzheimer's and ALS. Although there have been some dramatic results when Alzheimer's and ALS patients are tested for Lyme (and those with positive results put on an extended course of antibiotics), there is no absolute connection made at this time. What the studies did demonstrate, however, is that any older patient who has been diagnosed with either ALS or Alzheimer's, or is displaying some sort of motor-neuron disease, should be tested for Lyme so as not to ignore a medical problem that is reversible.

Since the older patient will be operating at a disadvantage, both because of the presentations of the illness and possibly because of age, it is very important that a family member or close friend enter into the therapeutic alliance with the doctor to assist in the history taking, asking pertinent questions and assisting the patient in following through on the doctor's recommendations.

Again, as with all other Lyme sufferers, do not accept ignorance or prejudice from your doctor. If you suggest Lyme and the physician refuses to consider it at all or to test for it, then a reevaluation of the doctor-patient relationship may be in order. Be aware that a major consideration in treating older patients is health coverage, whether the patient is with a commercial company or is on Medicare. The ability to pay for treatment once a diagnosis is made influences both the doctor and the senior citizen in accepting a diagnosis of Lyme.

"I DON'T HAVE LYME; I'M CRAZY!"

When Betty decided to retire to one of the great sprawling suburbs of Houston, within an easy drive of the Gulf of Mexico, she thought the golden time of life had finally arrived. Widowed for nearly ten years, the lively sixty-three-year-old had a modest fixed income, played tennis and golf regularly, traveled, and loved to sail with friends. In fact, it was sailing that brought her and her new husband together. Not only did they enjoy the rigors of hitting the open seas, they equally enjoyed hiking and camping the rugged hills in the western part of the state. It was on such a camping trip that Betty feels she must have been bitten by the infected tick.

"I never saw a rash, but then, I'm outside so much that I'm pretty tan most of the time. I know, I know, it's not good for the skin, but there you have it. I never noticed a tick bite. I wish I had," she says. "It would have made everything a whole lot easier."

Betty's symptoms began with a flu in September that left her weak, lethargic, and arthritic. She made the rounds of specialists, who each began by telling her that a woman her age had to expect these kinds of aches and pains, especially when doing "activities best left for the younger set." She began having problems with her hearing—it would come and go in one ear, alternating with a high-pitched squeal that would last only seconds yet leave her shaken.

Within weeks, her vision had deteriorated in her left eye, she could not move without intense pain, she was so dizzy she could not walk across a room, and she could barely lift her left arm. She again went through a battery of tests, which came up negative, and received the doctor's recommendation that she see a psychiatrist.

By that time Betty's personality had also undergone a change, and her husband thought a psychiatrist would not be a bad idea. From the outgoing, energetic, upbeat, and organized woman he had married, Betty had turned into a depressed, withdrawn woman whose mood swings ran the gamut from intense anger to a nearly catatonic state. What she didn't tell her husband was that she kept getting lost, forgot what she was going to say, and felt she was going crazy fast. On top of everything else, she developed bronchitis and her doctor put her on erythromycin, since she's allergic to penicillin. When she woke up one morning to find that her legs did not have the strength to hold her up, she was terrified.

Another round of doctor visits resulted in a diagnosis of acute Alzheimer's. The recommendation was either full-time nursing at home or admittance to a long-term care facility. It had been five months since her camping trip.

Betty's sister in Southern California badgered Betty's husband into asking for, and then demanding, a Lyme test. Betty tested negative, but her sister wasn't satisfied with the test in view of the antibiotic Betty had been taking for the bronchitis. A few weeks later, they requested a Western Blot that gave a faintly positive reading. Betty was put on an intravenous drug for the four weeks covered by her insurance plan. It was the beginning of a miraculous recovery.

"I actually began to get back to normal," she says. "I was still fatigued and still in a wheelchair, but my muscles began to work again, and I felt I was more in control of my emotions. Just as I was beginning to think I was on my way back to normal, we were told that my insurance coverage had hit its limit on all my tests and expensive treatments. I couldn't believe what I was hearing!"

We will get into the inequities and misguided protocols of insurance companies in chapter 17, but suffice it to say here that Betty had a battle on her hands. The only way to continue treatment, she was told, was for her doctor to diagnose something like a form of mental illness with complications so her office visits, counseling, and therapy could continue. She got back in touch with her sister, who put her in contact with a new doctor. After reviewing her case, this doctor agreed with the Lyme diagnosis and felt longer term treatment was indicated. He agreed to help her get the needed coverage.

Today Betty wears stronger glasses, still has aching joints on rainy days, and still wakes up in the morning in a "Lyme fog," but she is off antibiotics and walks regularly to get her strength and muscle tone back. And all this was made possible by declaring that she was "crazy," rather than sick with Lyme in a wheelchair, so her medical coverage could be continued.

OTHER TREATMENT CONSIDERATIONS

The cost of treatment is very much on the minds of older patients when they seek the help of a doctor. Particularly if they are on fixed incomes, the doctor's recommendations are measured against the backdrop of mortgage or rent payments, utility bills, and food bills. If patients must spend money on medicine, they won't have it to buy food—and they cannot get well without eating properly.

Then there is also the issue of compliance. There are two types of older patients—the ones who are obsessively compliant and will do everything the doctor says to the tiniest detail, and those who have no trust in the medical system and won't follow directions at all. As your parent's advocate, it is up to you either to hire a home health care nurse who can assist you with arranging meals and assuring that medications are taken or to handle this yourself.

In addition, the treatment of an older patient with Lyme must take into consideration how well the elder's liver is functioning and how well the kidneys are clearing the prescribed medication if the drug of choice is one that settles there. This will be determined through the doctor's history taking, physical examination, and supportive tests.

As the 76 million baby boomers join the millions who are already in the sixty-plus age bracket, doctors cannot afford to overlook a possible diagnosis of Lyme simply because the patient falls into a convenient age bracket. The advocate, the therapeutic alliance, and—in the case of the elders, the home-visiting nurse—will help to assure an accurate diagnosis of Lyme in the senior population, despite the challenges specific to this age group.

13.
Lyme Disease in Animals

What do a cat, a camel, and a giraffe have in common?

Not only are they the only four-legged animals that move legs on the opposite sides of the body at the same time, but despite their diverse geographical habitats they can all get Lyme disease. So can dogs, cattle, horses, rabbits, and many other animals. From Africa to Australia, from Europe to the United States, Lyme disease is hitting the animal population just as surely as the human.

Dr. Dorothy Feir, entomologist and professor of biology at Saint Louis University, points to Lyme disease as the cause of blindness in kangaroos at the Saint Louis Zoo. Cultures taken from the kidneys of the sick animals revealed the presence of the *Borrelia burgdorferi.* In Wisconsin, California, Connecticut, and Missouri, researchers and veterinarians are studying the transmission of Lyme disease among dairy and beef cattle, and even representatives from the Frank Perdue Company, in Salisbury, Maryland, are intensely vigilant in protecting the poultry industry from tick attack. Lyme disease is also on the minds of thousands of horse breeders across the country, because the chronic infection of one horse may result in the loss of hundreds of thousands of dollars.

While comparatively few people are concerned with Lyme in camels, millions are concerned about "man's best friend" because dogs are the prime animal victims of this disease worldwide. It should come as no surprise, since running through tall grass and wooded areas, rolling in fields, and crashing through underbrush rich with ticks is second nature to canines. This can throw their owners into a mass of confusion regarding diagnosis and treatment.

The spread of Lyme in animals parallels the spread to humans in endemic areas, since they are exposed to the same migratory birds and increasingly warmer climates due to the general global warming. In addition, they spend more time out of doors than most humans.

Like their human counterparts, animals generally get Lyme through the bite of an infected tick. As with humans, the diagnosis of Lyme must be a clinical one, as the same weaknesses in testing for antibodies apply. And like humans, these animals can quickly pass from early-stage to late-stage Lyme through a delay in diagnosis, which can render them chronically lame and arthritic.

Unlike most humans, however, animals may contract Lyme from the urine spray of other infected animals, do not usually display an EM rash, and respond to treatment more quickly and with fewer complications.

There are many questions surrounding animals—particularly house pets—and Lyme. The most common include: "Can humans get Lyme from their pets?" "What are the symptoms of Lyme in animals?" and "How can we prevent our pets from contracting Lyme disease?"

DOGS AND CATS AND LYME

Isabelle thought her vet was kidding when he said that all three of her beagles had Lyme disease. Sure they had slowed down (one didn't want to leave its stuffed circular bed), and they didn't seem to be eating properly, but she attributed that to the fact that they seemed to eat less in the fall.

But her dogs were prime candidates for the disease since they lived in an open field area bordered by woods, spent most of their time out-of-doors, and generally did not require daily brushing, which might have revealed either the ticks or the rash.

Dr. Barry Lissman, chairman of the Committee on Public Health and Regulatory Medicine for the New York State Veterinary Medical Society, was the first individual to discover and report clinical findings on both Rocky Mountain spotted fever and Lyme disease in dogs. Evaluating clinical findings of Lyme since 1983, Dr. Lissman won the Award for Outstanding Service to Veterinary Medicine in 1992 for his original work with Lyme disease. He feels that anyone living in Lyme-endemic areas should have their pets tested for Lyme, but they need to be aware that many animals can test positive yet not show any signs of Lyme.

Says Lissman, "Some animals may have, at some point, developed a resistance to the disease. The organism may have been lying dormant in the animal's body or the particular animal may have better immunity to the organism. Also, the number and kinds of ticks with which the animal has come in contact may play an important role in whether or not the animal will get the disease. Conversely, an animal may test negative and still have Lyme disease. A history of tick infestation or visits to endemic areas would be useful in a clinical diagnosis."

While cats can, and do, get Lyme disease, the incidence is much lower than for dogs. This is partially because they are primarily indoor animals, and they are better groomers than dogs, with their rough tongues acting as efficient "brooms" to rid themselves of ticks. If cats are bitten by ticks, the insects are more readily seen on the heads and even around the eye areas.

Just as in humans, Lyme disease can affect an animal's heart, eyes, nervous system, and kidneys. Humans may discuss "symptoms" of Lyme disease, but since animals can't speak, veterinarians prefer to refer to the "signs" of Lyme. In house pets, these include:

- Arthritis (lameness)
- Lethargy
- Sudden onset of severe pain
- Fever

- Loss of appetite
- Depression
- Other temperament and personality changes

Your veterinarian should be consulted as soon as you observe any of these changes in your pet so he can test for Lyme and rule out other diseases. Both dogs and cats respond quickly to an antibiotic regimen of three to four weeks if the disease is caught in the early stages. But the key to Lyme disease in house pets, as in humans, is prevention.

"Pets and humans should be checked for ticks once or twice a day and more thoroughly after a walk or run outdoors," says Dr. Lissman. "Outdoor areas should be treated periodically with an insecticide approved for use in kennels and/or outdoors. Tall grass, weeds, and brush in the area should be cut, and insecticide powders may help control ticks as will some of the newer Permethrin dips and sprays for dogs."

For both small dogs and cats, tick and flea collars recommended by your veterinarian are a good first step in protection. If you should see a tick on Rover or Fluffy, remove it with needle-nose tweezers—not your fingers, nail polish, or a match. As with any tick bite, care should be taken in removing the tick so as not to inadvertently squeeze the "poison" into the animal's system. The tick can then be saved for future identification by placing it in a small, closed container with a blade of grass and/or a piece of damp cotton.

Two laboratories have developed a vaccine that is designated for dogs. It is given as a series of two injections, three weeks apart, and must be boosted annually. Debate rages, however, on the efficacy of the vaccines currently available. They are not 100 percent foolproof, vets across the country caution, and owners should not be lulled into a false sense of security.

People cannot catch Lyme disease from their pets, and experts say it is unlikely that a tick that has attached itself to a pet will then "hop off" onto a human. Pet owners just need to be aware that their pets *can* bring ticks into the house, so a thorough daily examination would be in everyone's best interests.

LYME IN CATTLE

Despite the fact that Lyme disease is generally transmitted by a tick bite, there has been some concern that dairy workers could contract Lyme disease from the urine splash of infected cows. Indeed, this appears to be one method of transmission among herds of cattle, according to studies under way at both the University of Connecticut and the University of Wisconsin. Far from being a new manifestation, this came to the attention of researchers when massive cattle herd infection in the United Kingdom resulted in large numbers of animals having to be destroyed.

Although it has not yet been definitely proven, researchers say it is very possible and even likely for the *Borrelia* organism to pass from one cow to another through contaminated urine. Dairy cows are commonly housed closely together on concrete flooring, and it is common for them to sniff around each other's vulvas. But beyond this, when a cow urinates, particularly on a concrete floor, the splash can go as far as three feet, surely far enough to reach the cow's neighbor. (While the active particles of *Borrelia* are present in the urine, once the urine has dried the organism is dead.)

By extension, this theory of infection would support Dr. Willy Burgdorfer's contention that he contracted Lyme disease from the urine of infected rabbits while he was performing research into Rocky Mountain spotted fever.

Another concern regarding Lyme disease and cattle is whether the organism can be passed to humans via cows' milk or, in the case of beef cattle, through infected meat. Researchers say that, at this time, there is no evidence to suggest that the spirochetes can survive the pasteurization process or any type of cooking process, because heat destroys these organisms as it does other bacteria.

HORSES

Whether a horse costs $4,000 or $400,000, unrecognized and/or untreated Lyme disease can result not only in chronic physical pain for the animal but in emotional devastation and financial burdens for the owner.

Like humans and small pets, horses display a variety of symptoms that may signal Lyme disease and should send up a red flag to call the veterinarian. These include:

- Lameness
- Swelling, pain, or stiffness in the joints of the legs
- Uncoordination
- Fatigue
- Skin hypersensitivity resulting in refusal to be saddled
- Weight loss
- Behavior/attitude changes (i.e., lethargy, aggression, diminished ambition/performance—sometimes referred to as "being a little off")
- Nerve tremors
- Fetal resorptions/abortions
- Nephritis (inflammation of the kidneys)
- Foundering due to laminitis (inflammation of the hoof)

Again, as with humans and other animals, the diagnosis of Lyme disease must be a clinical one, particularly if the blood tests show up negative.

Dr. Jonathan Palmer, an equine specialist at the University of Pennsylvania, says that the important guidepost for diagnosing Lyme in horses is observance of the physical signs of the disease. "It is possible for a horse to be infected by a tick bite and have a negative test result because the animal has not accumulated antibodies yet. It is also possible for a horse to have a positive antibody titer test and be able to fight off the organism without getting the disease. Up to 60 percent of horses will have antibody titers if they live in a Lyme-endemic area, but very few of these will have Lyme disease."

Dr. Palmer says that the industry is looking to depend on the developing reliability of the PCR testing techniques for establishing whether a horse actually has Lyme or not. Until then, a local history of tick infestation, signs of illness, and response to antibiotics remain the diagnostic guidelines.

In treating equine Lyme, veterinarians must also consider the types of antibiotics used, as some common ones can cause undesirable side effects. For example, Tribrissen (a sulfa drug) is not always effective, and doxycycline, which is used in both humans and canines, can produce fatal arrhythmia (abnormal heartbeats) in horses.

Currently, there is no Lyme vaccine available for animals other than dogs.

III.

GETTING

TREATMENT

AND SUPPORT

Doctors pour drugs of which they know little, to cure diseases of which they know less, into human beings of whom they know nothing.

—VOLTAIRE

14.

Treatment: The Long and Short of It

I have had two cancers and Lyme disease. With all the pain and suffering that goes along with cancer, I still beat them. I'd trade my Lyme disease for two more cancers any day.

—Cindy M., twenty-eight years old

The definitive treatment for Lyme disease is best expressed by a statement made by Dr. Jorge Benach, professor of pathology specializing in Lyme at the State University of New York, Stony Brook, during a conference in December 1992. He said, "Nothing I say can be taken as gospel truth. It is subject to change, it will very likely change, and will probably be challenged."

Even though it has been a dozen years since those words were uttered, they remain true for a variety of reasons. With all that the medical experts and researchers have learned about the Lyme disease spirochete, with all that they know but are ignoring, and with all that is changing, *there is still no definitive and standard treatment protocol for Lyme disease at present.* This is primarily because the choice of medication used and the dosage prescribed vary for each person based on factors such as the age of the patient, the level and type of infection, the potential for co-infections, and the patient's history of drug tolerance and immunosuppressants. And while that might seem like common sense and good medical practice, it remains the crux of the controversy that has polarized doctors, involved insurance companies, and sent ailing patients on lengthy searches for relief. As one patient who has three immediate family members suffering with Lyme said, "What is the problem? Cancer patients don't have to fight for chemotherapy and everyone knows *that* has bad side effects. Why do Lyme patients have to fight for treatment?"

Why, indeed? If we operate from the belief that patients want to get well, and doctors want to heal, it would seem a straightforward matter that doctors would prescribe whatever medication works for as long as it takes to eradicate the symptoms of the disease, thereby assuring that the patient is cured.

As we have already seen, however, nothing is straightforward and simple with Lyme disease, and treatment is no exception.

The controversy arises primarily around the length of time a patient is medicated. Many university-based researchers, who are accustomed to performing controlled studies both in and out of laboratories, maintain that Lyme disease should be "cured" in fourteen to twenty-eight days of antibiotic therapy. It has been proven, however, that antibiotics that seem to work well at eradicating bacteria in the test tube don't perform in the same manner when injected into the human body.

The aggressive clinicians who are swamped with hurting and degenerating Lyme patients maintain that swift and aggressive antibiotic therapy should be continued for as long as the patient has Lyme disease symptoms. This stand is based not only on numerous published research papers detailing the ineffectiveness of short-term therapy for this uniquely potent organism but on the results from literally thousands of Lyme patients who have been treated for varied lengths of time.

Finally, there is a third and growing segment composed of both researchers and clinicians who are weighing all available published data on Lyme with epidemiological evidence and patient histories and are taking a more "middle-of-the-road" approach. They may be aggressively diagnosing Lyme and beginning treatment, yet they are cautious to reevaluate each patient individually as treatment progresses, extending treatment when necessary and providing their patients with adjunctive therapies to boost the body's immune system.

It is these doctors who point to precedents set by the treatment of such things as tuberculosis (another disease with a slow replication rate), which is routinely *initially* treated for six to nine months with multiple antibiotics, and teenage acne, which is routinely treated with antibiotics—uncontroversially—for two years. This has prompted many physicians to say, "If we can treat zits with antibiotics for two years, what is the problem with treating patients ill with Lyme disease for longer than twenty-one days?"

This singling out of Lyme becomes even more confusing when a venerable entity like the *New England Journal of Medicine* publishes an article in the fall of 2002 detailing an experimental treatment for hepatitis C of weekly injections of a long-acting form of interferon—known to cause liver damage—for a minimum of forty-eight weeks, resulting in a cure of just 56 percent of the patients. Despite the fact that the drug's side effects include depression, fatigue, and loss of hair, the drug was welcomed by such learned researchers as Dr. Michael Fried of the University of North Carolina at Chapel Hill because one of the drug's advantages is that doctors can tell by the twelfth week which patients are responding well. "This means that physicians can create an alternate treatment plan for patients who do not show any response by week twelve," he said.

Finally, controversy surrounds the behavior of the organism itself, which has thrown the meaning of the "cure" into contention. It has been documented that the *Borrelia burgdorferi* spirochete can not only change its protein "appearance," once disseminated in the body, but that it can also "hide" from antibiotics within human cells, thus evading eradication by antibiotics. And, as we discussed earlier, some of the newest research has shown that the spirochete can actually adopt a cystlike form to evade an antibiotic evasion until the coast is clear. For these reasons, this spirochete, like the syphilis spirochete, can go into a dormant period wherein the patient may be free from symptoms, only to relapse when the spirochete flares again.

Although academics say that a patient is "cured" of Lyme after a specified number of days of treatment, regardless of the symptoms that remain, the majority of clinicians who treat Lyme agree that a patient is not "cured" unless he or she is totally symptom-free for at least two months.

Regardless of a doctor's position on length of therapy, the initial evaluation of the patient's need for antibiotics is based on a classification of symptoms by stages. Depending on the severity of symptoms and the stage of the disease, the doctor will make a recommendation as to whether the patient needs oral antibiotics or intravenous antibiotics, and which type of antibiotics to use.

THE STAGES OF LYME DISEASE

There are now five recognized stages of Lyme disease: the tick bite, early localized, early disseminated, late disseminated, and chronic. Like most anything else involving Lyme disease, the following chart for gauging the development of the disease is simply a guideline. It is important to remember two things. First, because each person's body is different, one person may pass from the early stage to the late disseminated stage within a few weeks, while another person will take months or even years to progress to that stage.

Second, especially in the early disseminated, late disseminated, and chronic stages, the symptoms do overlap and may vary. One person might have cardiac symptoms associated with early disseminated Lyme, yet be in a chronic stage for everything else.

Due to the overwhelming number of patients who display chronic symptoms for varying periods of time, the chronic stage is included in the chart, but see chapter 15 for a discussion of chronic Lyme. Since the tick bite may be a precursor to infection but does not lead to Lyme in every case, we will address this stage following the treatment protocols. For purposes of discussion, we will initially look at just three of the stages of Lyme disease.

STAGES AND SYMPTOMS OF LYME DISEASE

Early Localized	Disseminated		Chronic
	EARLY	LATE	
EM rash	Headache	Severe headaches/ migraines	Migraines
	Joint pains	Crippling arthritis	Arthritis
	Body aches	Swollen joints	
	Night sweats	Heart blockage	Loss of libido
	Sensitivity to light, sound, touch	Hypersensitivity to light, sound, touch	
	Migratory pains	Crippling migratory pains	
	Bell's palsy		
	Fatigue	Severe fatigue	Fatigue
	Heart palpitations	Optic neuritis and increased eye complications	
	Swollen glands		
	Stiff neck		
	Worsening of asthmatic symptoms	Seizures	
		Nosebleeds	Muscle weakness
	Disorientation	Memory loss	
	Lyme fog	Lyme fog	Lyme fog
	Conjunctivitis	Dyslexic reversals	Dyslexia
	Sleep disturbances	Sleep disturbances, nightmares	
		Abnormal MRI, CAT scan, EEG, CSF	

COMMONLY USED ANTIBIOTICS

The physicians will evaluate a patient's symptoms against the backdrop of the three primary stages before prescribing an antibiotic treatment. However, there is no universally effective antibiotic for treating Lyme disease at this time. Although I will describe the types of antibiotics used, I will not outline prescribed amounts as these not only can change but are up to the individual physicians to determine. Suffice it to say that the amounts normally prescribed to attack the Lyme disease spirochete are usually much greater than those normally prescribed for a common bacterial infection.

There are four primary types of antibiotics used to fight Lyme disease, although only one of the classifications was developed with Lyme disease in mind. The others are all general-use, broad-spectrum antibiotics.

The tetracyclines   These include doxycycline and minocycline. While these have been somewhat effective for the early stage of Lyme, many doctors feel that they are ineffective for later stages. Minocycline seems to have shown effectiveness in penetrating the cerebrospinal fluid as well as ocular tissues and possessing intrinsic anti-inflammatory properties, and it is often easier on the gastrointestinal tract. Some clinicians have been able to treat some patients with neurologic Lyme with this agent. A dose of 300 to 400 mg per day of doxycycline may be needed to treat adequately for CNS disease.

The tetracyclines are not recommended for pregnant women or children under the age of twelve, as they can cause the malformation and staining of developing teeth, as well as some blood problems.

The penicillins   Amoxicillin has proven to be a good all-around treatment for early-stage Lyme and, in combinations with other antibiotics, for late stages. In addition, it is the only drug of choice at this time for a pregnant woman, as it causes relatively few side effects. It can be administered orally or intravenously.

Sometimes the drug probenecid is prescribed in conjunction with amoxicillin as a booster or facilitator for the antibiotic. It is not recommended for use in children or pregnant women, however, or in anyone with a history of kidney problems.

The macrolides   Erythromycin causes the fewest side effects, but at the same time has proven ineffective as a Lyme antibiotic when used by itself. It may be used in combination with another drug. The advanced azalides, azithromycin (Zithromax) and clarithromycin (Biaxin), have been used for Lyme disease treatment. So far in clinical trials, they seem to be more effective than some other antibiotics in treating late stage Lyme, particularly when neurological problems are involved. Some preliminary work regarding the administering of Zithromax intravenously is being done. At the time of this writing, these two drugs are administered orally.

Because Zithromax and Biaxin are particularly potent, they have an impact on the intestinal tract and must be counterbalanced with nutritional adjunctive therapies (see page 174) to keep the body on an even keel.

The cephalosporins The antibiotics from this group are generally second- or third-generation derivatives of other drugs, designed to penetrate a greater number of tissues more effectively. Ceftin and Suprax are the oral antibiotics; Rocephin and Claforan are the two antibiotics commonly used in IV therapy.

Rocephin has, in some cases, produced gallbladder symptoms, particularly in women. Therefore, Claforan is quickly becoming the drug of choice. As with Zithromax and Biaxin, adjunctive nutritional therapies are recommended to prevent diarrhea and stomach cramps.

There are a couple of other drugs that doctors may prescribe on an individual basis that include Primaxin, ciprofloxacin, Bactrim, and metronidazole (see chapter 15).

If a patient goes to the doctor with an EM rash (early stage), the general consensus is to treat that patient for three to four weeks with amoxicillin. At this point in the course of the disease, aggressive treatment will usually eliminate any further symptoms and dissemination of the disease. The key is to treat early, aggressively, and for a sufficient length of time in order to effect a "cure"—defined as the complete resolution of the disease process or state.

The disseminated stages of Lyme are more difficult to treat because the disease has been carried throughout the patient's body and the spirochete has had an opportunity to establish "hiding" places. If a person has the EM rash and some of the symptoms of early disseminated Lyme, the general choice of treatment would be an oral antibiotic for an initial period of at least four to six weeks. At the end of the initial treatment cycle, the doctor should evaluate the patient for continuing symptoms and signs of infection.

If a doctor sees a patient with late disseminated Lyme, or a large overlap of symptoms, including neurological impairment, he or she will likely put the patient immediately on an IV therapy regimen for an initial phase of four to six weeks, followed by evaluation of the need for continuing antibiotics. At that time, depending upon the patient's symptoms, the doctor may extend IV therapy for another few weeks, or place the patient on oral antibiotics until he or she is symptom free.

During ongoing antibiotic treatment, the doctor should do monthly blood work on an "orals" patient, and weekly or bimonthly blood work on an "IV" patient. This will allow the doctor to look for abnormalities in white blood cells as well as monitor the patient's liver functions.

ADJUNCTIVE THERAPIES

One of the concerns patients express is that they have heard that heavy or long-term antibiotic use will destroy the body's immune system and render their bodies defenseless against other infections. This criticism is also leveled by some of the medical critics of longer-term antibiotic treatment.

No one can give a guarantee regarding any medical treatment, and any medication can cause side effects. Based on long-term antibiotic treatments of such diseases as tuberculosis, urinary tract infections, acne, and children's chronic ear infections, however, there is little reason to suspect that antibiotic treatment of longer than several months' duration will destroy the body or cause subsequent infections to be immune to other antibiotics.

What antibiotics do, however, is diminish the flora in the intestinal tract, which must be replaced to keep the body in balance. For that reason, any Lyme patient who is on a strong antibiotic regimen should pay particular attention to diet and nutrition in order to counteract the effects of a disrupted biological balance, ward off yeast infections, and rebuild the body's immune system. This will be dealt with in detail in chapter 18, "Diet and Nutrition."

Other adjunctive therapies, including aerobic exercise, will be discussed in chapter 19.

THE JARISH-HERXHEIMER REACTION

Many Lyme patients who are in the early disseminated stage and beyond will, once placed on antibiotics, experience a period of worsening symptoms—sometimes dramatically—soon after the antibiotic regimen has begun. This is called the Jarish-Herxheimer reaction and is not only to be expected but is actually a good sign that the drug is hitting its target.

Sometimes interpreted by unknowing doctors and patients alike as an allergic reaction to the antibiotic, the Herxheimer (as it is commonly called) occurs when the spirochete, attacked by the drug, gives off toxins and causes the immune system to overreact. It's as though a bomb were dropped on the spirochete, breaking it into ten pieces. Suddenly the body has to fight ten times as hard for a short period of time to eliminate it.

There may be varying degrees of Herxheimer, with additional rashes, headaches, chills, fevers, and lowered blood pressure. *This is a normal and expected reaction.* Do not stop taking your medication should you experience this worsening of symptoms. Do contact your physician, however, and let him or her decide whether you are having a Herxheimer or a real allergic reaction.

Generally, the longer the time between the initial dose of medicine and the Herxheimer, the more disseminated the disease and the longer the treatment may be needed. A Herxheimer reaction can last from two days to two weeks, so a doctor's support is critical.

PULSE THERAPY

Pulse therapy refers to a system whereby a patient gets on a cycle of taking an antibiotic (either orally or intravenously) for several days, then discontinuing for several days. This is called "pulsing."

The theory behind pulse therapy is this: antibiotics kill the spirochete only while it is actively replicating. Not only does the *Borrelia burgdorferi* replicate very slowly, it can become dormant and evade the antibiotics. Thus pulse therapy is based on the idea that the organism will be active and replicate while the patient is off the antibiotics, then can be zapped with a dose when the patient is back on. This is not very different from the pulse therapy used to treat cancer patients going through chemotherapy, and is sometimes used by doctors with patients who have not responded well to other treatments, or who have been on antibiotics for a long time and are still symptomatic.

While it is not recommended or used by all doctors treating Lyme, it has credible advocates. Like any other Lyme treatment, this must be up to the physician and decided on a case-by-case basis. Continuing research should determine the long-term effectiveness of pulse therapy.

COMBINATION THERAPY

Until such time as a Lyme disease–specific antibiotic is developed, many physicians have found that combining two, and sometimes three, of the currently used drugs increases their ability to damage the spirochete and eliminate it from the system. This method utilizes the strength of each antibiotic for a synergistic effect and has become more common in treating patients with disseminated and neurologic Lyme symptoms, and in treating those patients with multiple tick-borne co-infections. The only real drawback for patients in combination therapy is that they must pay close attention to diet and nutritional supplements in order to combat the effects of megadosages on the gastrointestinal tract and the balance of flora in the system (see chapter 18).

THE TICK BITE AND PROPHYLACTIC TREATMENT

Six-year-old Jenny lives in Saint Paul, Minnesota, and belongs to a family of campers. At least they *were* campers—until Lyme disease brought Jenny's eighteen-year-old brother and her mother to their swollen knees. So when Jenny came home from a friend's house after spending the night and her mother noticed a suspicious dot on the back of her leg during her bath, you can imagine the concern it generated throughout the small family.

Recognizing the tick and removing it carefully, Jenny's mother called the pediatrician and asked that Jenny be put on antibiotics immediately. When the pediatrician assessed the disseminated symptoms suffered by Jenny's mother and brother and acknowledged the fact that they live in a Lyme-endemic area and that Jenny didn't know how long the tick had been attached to her, he agreed.

His decision to put Jenny on amoxicillin for three weeks assured that, should the tick be infected, Jenny would be safe and cured without suffering the same debilitating problems her family members faced. Yet his decision is one that is debated among medical professionals across the country, particularly in the face of the NIH's new campaign to make physicians and the public aware that overuse of antibiotics leads to drug-resistant bacteria. There are no attempts made, however, to outline the exceptions—and Lyme should be a huge exception.

In a paper published by the *New England Journal of Medicine* during the summer of 1992, a study jointly sponsored by the Universities of Colorado and Pennsylvania, Johns Hopkins, and Yale revealed that treating tick bites prophylactically was not only more efficient health-wise but was more cost-effective as well.

This study evaluated three alternatives: (1) empirically treat all patients with two weeks of antibiotics; (2) treat only those in whom the EM rash develops; and (3) treat only those who display an EM rash and have a positive blood test. The results showed that since nearly 50 percent of the people bitten by ticks do not have or remember a rash, by the time other symptoms developed or blood tests were positive, the disease had disseminated throughout their systems and thus presented major treatment and recovery problems. Apart from the common sense of disease prevention, the study also showed that it was more cost-effective all the way around to treat a tick bite for two weeks than to have to institute either oral or intravenous therapy for a longer period of time (not to mention the cost of time lost from work, school, and other activities).

Dr. Robert Femia is a new breed of physician. At forty-one, this director of emergency services for Greenwich Hospital is not only board certified in emergency medicine but also holds an M.B.A. from Indiana-Wesleyan. He oversees a group of ten physicians ranging in age from thirty-two to sixty-one in one of the country's more Lyme-endemic areas. His approach to medicine is common sense—an attitude, he says, that is more prevalent among those who work in hospital emergency rooms because of the nature of their specialty.

"I can't say that every single time someone comes in with a tick bite they'll go home with antibiotics, because every case is different. But this is an endemic area. Let's be practical; I'm not going to rely on the twenty-hour rule. We can send the tick off for testing and we can discuss antibiotics with the patient and treat prophylactically, but to do nothing at all is unacceptable," Femia says. "ER docs tend to be more comfortable in an arena where decisions are made before everything is studied and all the results are in. It's a matter of weighing risks and benefits. You can't breathe? First, I'll help you breathe better and *then* we'll find out why you can't breathe.

"We have a working agreement in the ER and the docs here are pretty savvy. They know that the ELISA and Western Blot aren't usually definitive, and they feel comfortable making clinical judgments because that is the inherent nature of ER medicine. I have seen what Lyme disease can do and I get concerned when someone is dogmatic about treatment. This is an area that has very soft boundaries—there are no black and whites. One of the other things we do is hold community meetings to follow up with the doctors in our area so we can see what impact our treatment in the ER has had, or not had.

"Should everyone treat a tick bite? I wouldn't presume to say," Femia says. "But for me, if I take a tick off someone in this area where forty-three percent of the ticks are infected, I'll give them ten days of antibiotics and send the tick to the lab. I ask myself, 'Is this going to help or hurt the patient?' and go on from there. I'd rather err on the side of preventing a terrible illness from taking hold."

There are still many physicians who do not want to put anyone on an antibiotic unless given irrefutable evidence of infection. There are also those who would probably like to put the entire population of the United States on antibiotics, "just in case." But the majority—particularly those who have treated patients suffering with serious Lyme manifestations—recommend that tick bites in Lyme-endemic areas be treated swiftly and aggressively.

Frankly, *that* is the kind of doctor I would take *my* child to if she were bitten by a tick in this endemic area.

POTENTIALLY DANGEROUS THERAPIES

Any time the public is faced with a disease that causes tremendous distress and is difficult to cure, there exists the possibility of dangerous experimental therapies cropping up as desperate people look for relief. Lyme disease is no exception.

Two experimental therapies that have been tried by patients

are malaria therapy and hydrogen peroxide therapy. Those who have tried them say that they were not worth the pain and suffering and did not result in the hoped-for cure.

Malaria therapy is based upon the idea that the spirochete cannot live in a high-temperature setting. Therefore, it is of interest that the standard treatment period of two to four weeks was originally based on comparing the behavior of the Lyme spirochete to that of another spirochetal disease, syphilis. It has since been proven, however, that they don't follow the same initial theory of behavior, but some ideas die hard. This group of doctors acts like a dog who won't relinquish his bone simply because it's his. The difference is that the dog can eventually go off with no ill effects. Doctors who refuse to recognize that Lyme disease can remain active in the system for much longer than the arbitrary two to four weeks are dangerous to their patients.

They are dangerous because they haven't reviewed current literature; because their obstinacy can cause complications and further illness in their patients; and because they influence other, less informed doctors who decide to "go with the flow" rather than read, study, and decide for themselves.

Another influence on the doctors who obstinately maintain that Lyme disease "should be cured in two to four weeks" is that they are often hired by insurance companies that depend on medical professionals not only to advise them on disease treatments but also to justify minimal coverages. This is not to say that all doctors who advocate brief treatment for Lyme are on insurance company payrolls, but some of the major insurance providers in the country today have purposely sought out the most conservative medical element, even in the face of contradictory evidence (more on insurance companies in chapter 17).

There are dozens of studies showing that four weeks of antibiotic therapy gives incomplete resolution of symptoms, or permits the patient to relapse. These include documentation from reputable and distinguished researchers detailing how active spirochetes have been cultured from the bodies of patients who have completed antibiotic therapies for six months' duration or longer (see the bibliography).

In fact, the late Dr. Paul Lavoie, noted rheumatologist and Lyme disease pioneer, said, "I have found evidence for persistent infection in improved patients with ongoing antibiotic therapy of a few years.

"This supports the concept that a bacteriologic cure is not easily achieved by current therapies and that we must not dismiss our patients' complaints following even very prolonged therapy. We must keep an open mind."

There are also a dozen or more published articles and reports showing that longer therapy can give progressive relief, fewer relapses and/or retreatments, and control resurgent symptoms (see the bibliography).

And in a study completed by the Committee on Infectious Diseases for the American Academy of Pediatrics, Chairman Dr. Stanley A. Plotkin stated: "If all symptoms have resolved, no further therapy is indicated. If symptoms persist, continued therapy is necessary until they have been resolved. Relapses can occur, requiring treatment with the same or other antibiotics."

In addition, the National Institutes of Health, in a special publication on Lyme disease, concludes: "Later manifestations of Lyme disease are more difficult to treat, sometimes requiring longer and more intensive use of oral antibiotics or intravenous antibiotics, particularly in patients with central nervous system involvement. The efficacy of long courses of antibiotic therapy remains to be demonstrated and needs further study."

Perhaps during the course of the NIH's million-dollar-plus study on chronic Lyme disease and its toll on Lyme victims, more doctors will take a moderate position, and gradually a consensus will be achieved.

Dr. Daniel Cameron, an internist and Lyme researcher in Mount Kisco, New York, is accustomed to being on the firing line. A former academic researcher who headed the National Task Force on Aging, Cameron the clinician, who has published and presented more than thirty scientific papers and serves on the boards of the International Lyme and Associated Diseases Society and the Lyme Disease Association, has a reputation for meticulously challenging researchers at national and international conferences who present papers and theories unsupported by the latest literature. His position represents a growing third "camp" in the Lyme disease medical arena.

"I base treatment on the literature, not the position of my peers. For this reason, I find I am in the middle ground regarding treatment, not diagnosis. I make a diagnosis on clinical grounds. There are many diseases in medicine which we treat even though there may be a low probability that the patient has them, but we do it because, if untreated, they will progress to something much more serious. I feel Lyme disease falls into this category."

Cameron is not sitting back on his heels, simply waiting for the literature to evolve. He established the Lyme Project in 1997 to amass a national Lyme Surveillance Database and has conducted a series of clinical trials on various aspects of Lyme. Currently, he is conducting the Re-treatment Study, a double-blind clinical trial designed to compare the efficacy of using amoxicillin, as compared to other drugs, in re-treating Lyme patients who are experiencing problems after having been successfully treated for Lyme at least once before. Anyone interested in finding out more about Dr. Cameron's Re-treatment Study or his other projects can contact his office or visit his website (see appendix C).

The bottom line is that studies will eventually give rise to treatment protocols that will be standardized, with enough flexibility to allow for individual patient response, and the controversy over Lyme treatment will die down. But people who are ill now cannot wait for those studies. Every day that passes for patients with untreated Lyme disease may seal their futures into a pattern of chronic and debilitating illness.

If you have been treated for Lyme for four weeks and still feel ill, you should go back to the doctor and make this clear. Again, do not accept avoidance from your doctor. But remember, too, that your doctor won't know the four-week cure didn't work unless you go back and say so.

If you did not get an early diagnosis and aggressive treatment for Lyme disease, there is a possibility that you will continue to feel various effects of the disease for months and years to come. Fortunately, chronic Lyme disease has not only finally been recognized by the CDC and the NIH, but it is also the focus of a study to assess the damage it causes and to develop a successful treatment protocol.

15.

Chronic Lyme Disease

Modern physicians have mastered admirably the power of the latest scientific medicine. To excel at the art of healing requires the same systematic discipline. Healing begins with caring. So does civilization.

—Bill Moyers, *Healing and the Mind*

There is nothing worse than fighting a dual battle for credibility and wellness only to find that the organisms that have invaded your body will be with you for some time to come, keeping you in that purgatory of never feeling quite like your old self, yet lacking the weight of immediate crisis. Perhaps this is one of the reasons why, for so many years, those Lyme patients whose bodies spun them almost immediately into a disseminated stage, or who slid into a late disseminated stage because they couldn't get a timely diagnosis, were never taken seriously.

But chronic Lyme disease *is* serious. And now, after thousands of patients and hundreds of knowledgeable doctors and researchers have documented millions of instances where the spirochete lies dormant, evades antibiotics, and regenerates itself at its own whim, the official institutions of the NIH and CDC—as well as many formerly resistant academics—acknowledge the existence of chronic Lyme and the need to treat it in a multimodal approach. This is a positive change that has occurred over the years.

The term "chronic Lyme disease" is usually used to describe patients with an active infection of at least a year or more who have persistent major neurologic, arthritic, or constitutional manifestations even after antibiotic treatment. These patients are more likely to have a higher burden of infection, weaker immune systems, possibly a more virulent or resistant strain of the bacteria, and they may also be co-infected. Chances are that the neurological symptoms of Lyme play a significant role in keeping the chronic Lyme patient from feeling good.

Chronic Lyme disease is also used to describe those people who, after having been treated for an active infection of long duration, continue to suffer the lingering and damaging neurological and physical effects of the illness.

Martha, an accountant, is a perfect example. The thirty-two-year-old runner contracted Lyme while on a May vacation visiting family in Houston. When she woke up one morning with a pounding headache and a blotchy rash across her face, she attributed it to pushing her training miles in anticipation of her first marathon. Then came the flu-like illness, fever, stiff neck, and joint pain. "See?" her well-meaning parents told her. "You've been pushing too hard. No human was meant to run fifteen miles at a clip without something breaking down." By the time Martha visited her parents' doctor days later, she was still feeling "off" and exhausted, but the rash was gone. "Looking back on it now," she says, "that was the day my good health hit the road in the opposite direction."

For the next year, Martha's body fell apart. Back home in Virginia, she made the rounds of doctors as her legs began to fail, then her eyesight wavered, and then she lost strength in her arms and hands. She could no longer concentrate—essential when you are an accountant. When she asked about Lyme disease, she was told that Texas and Virginia don't have Lyme ticks. She was, they said, exhibiting all the signs of multiple sclerosis. "I was shocked and devastated," says Martha. "By Christmas, I was in a wheelchair. My parents rented out their house and came up to live with me so I could be close to my doctors. I was looking down a long, dark tunnel, ending in . . . well, let's put it this way—I know myself and I wouldn't have just waited to waste away. I was already in a lot of pain. I just wanted it to end. Then my sister came to visit."

Martha's sister, who lived in Nantucket where Lyme has invaded a high percentage of the households, was shocked when she saw Martha's deterioration. She called her own doctor and navigated the waters of getting Martha tested. Martha tested positive on five bands of the Western Blot and began treatment. Because of the severity of her condition and the length of time she had been infected, she was started on IV antibiotics immediately and stayed on them for four months. "It was unbelievable!" says Martha. "After about ten days I had a horrible Herxheimer, and then every day, it got a little better." Off the IV, she relapsed and her doctor put her on oral antibiotics, which she stayed on for another six months.

Now, three years later, she is finally off antibiotics, but has flares of Lyme symptoms around the time of her menstrual period. She has to support herself with several part-time book-keeping jobs since she cannot put in a full day of work as an accountant anymore. Her running days, she says, are over. Chronic Lyme runs her life now. "I look at pictures of me from just five years ago and it seems like I'm looking at a stranger," she says.

Once covered with the blanket term "post–Lyme syndrome," chronic Lyme gained independent "respectability" during the late 1990s and is now the focus of a number of studies being funded by the NIH and the NIAID, including the Chronic Lyme Disease Study being conducted at Columbia University under the direction of Dr. Brian Fallon, director of the Lyme Disease Research Program.

THE CHRONIC LYME DISEASE STUDY

There are five main questions that the Chronic Lyme Study is designed to answer, says Fallon. "First, do patients with persistent symptoms benefit from a repeated ten-week course of IV antibiotic therapy? Second, using state-of-the-art imaging to investigate the brain, do patients have a problem in the nerve cells of their brain, in the blood vessels, or both? Third, are there markers that predict who will benefit from therapy and who will not? Fourth, do the brain-imaging abnormalities improve with time, and if so, is the time line of improvement similar to the time line of neuropsychological testing? And finally, when they are off antibiotics entirely, do these chronic Lyme patients improve over time, stay the same, or relapse?"

Fallon's study, which is scheduled to continue into 2005, provides free brain imaging, performed at Columbia University and Columbia Presbyterian Hospital, in addition to a host of other tests done in cooperation with investigators at other institutions. Fallon says he is hopeful that this study, like his previous study of children with chronic Lyme who still suffered cognitive defects, will pave the way for understanding chronic Lyme disease and the creation of effective treatment protocols. (See appendix C for further information on eligibility and contacts.)

"There is finally an awareness concerning chronic Lyme disease that people's lives can be devastated and that troubling and continuing cases do exist," says Fallon. "How do we help these people? That's still the burning question."

It's a question—and a controversy—that a number of entities hope will move closer to an answer with the opening of the Columbia Lyme Center, the first of its kind in the country. "Just like people go to the Mayo clinic to find out what's wrong when everyone else has failed them, we envision a place where people can find answers and hope," says Fallon.

THE CHRONIC CONTROVERSY

Although the existence of chronic Lyme disease is no longer in controversy, the treatment for it remains a point of contention among medical professionals who take stabs at attempting to draw a line between active-infection illness and the residual effects of having one's body beaten down. While some physicians treat chronic Lyme until the symptoms disappear completely, utilizing a protocol that may include intravenous antibiotics followed by orals for a period of time, others argue that chronic Lyme is related more to the need to build up the body's immune system and physical abilities than it is to active infection.

The Chronic Lyme Study and several others which are being funded by the NIH and the Lyme Disease Association are paving the way for a wider spectrum of treatment. In the meantime, many physicians are adopting an individualized treatment approach that may include antibiotic therapy as well as other adjunctive therapies to help a patient regain his or her strength and health (see chapters 18 and 19).

Dealing with chronic Lyme disease, as with any chronic illness, can be disheartening and frustrating. Some of the frustration comes from pain, and some from comparing the person you were with the limitations the illness has placed upon you now. But a more limited life doesn't have to be one devoid of richness. As a writer and producer for most of my life, I have seen the value of editing a manuscript, a television segment, or an individual work. When you edit, you cut out the extraneous and focus on the important elements. This is true of coping with chronic Lyme disease as well. All you need is a little life editing:

- Enjoy your loved ones, friends, and an activity that lights a passion in you.
- Distract yourself from the illness. We all have aches and pains from living; if you dwell on each one, they will grow in size and overtake your life. Get involved in doing something for someone who needs *your* help.
- Inform yourself, as any good medical consumer would, on the latest studies and advances that might influence your wellness.
- Take pride in your appearance, your ability to design a good nutrition and exercise program, and the small accomplishments of each day.

Most of our lives can use a little EDITing. You will just have a head start.

If you have been diagnosed with Lyme disease in either the disseminated or chronic stages and require intravenous (IV) medication, it may sound scary. No need to conjure up scenarios of being restricted to bed with a bottle hanging from a stand. In truth, today, most IV patients have a choice: remain at home during certain times of the day or go about your job or school activities, and conduct life as usual—with the help of a growing new breed of health care professionals.

16.

Home Care Systems: The Modern House Call

When television's beloved Dr. Marcus Welby routinely stopped by a patient's home to check on her progress and support systems and help solve any myriad of personal problems, grandparents throughout the country nodded, remembering their own kindly doctors from bygone days. During the mid-twentieth century, however, medical care became "hospital centered." Expensive and bulky diagnostic equipment, sterile techniques, and growing populations made it nearly impossible for physicians to routinely visit sick patients at home.

With the average age of Americans continuing to rise and with an increase in chronic illnesses and decrease in insurance coverage, a new era in health care is sweeping in, along with some pretty startling numbers. According to the Bureau of Labor Statistics, by 2008 nearly three million new health care jobs will be added and the fastest growing category is in the area of home health care services, with a jump of 76 percent.

Although physicians who visit homes are still in the minority, a new kind of health professional is once more bringing medical treatment to the home—and the office, and the school—and is sometimes even meeting patients on the road. This is of particular interest to Lyme patients in any stage requiring intravenous therapy since it means that they can continue their lives, for the most part, surrounded by family and engaging in most of the activities they normally enjoy.

Home health care companies have a history stretching back to visiting nurse associations. Modern chronic disease treatments, including those for Lyme, are now often being handled in the home by a specifically trained nurse supported by a team of pharmacists, clinicians, and other specialists who work in tandem with the patient's doctor. This nurse will visit the IV patient weekly, change dressings, take a weekly history of progress and/or complaints, assess the supplies, and lend a human touch to the getting-well process. This approach to therapy is often the first time many people have contact with "at home" care.

When Jack, a corporate attorney in Atlanta, was told he had late disseminated Lyme disease and needed to be on IV therapy, he thought his life was over. "I was already trying to hang on while my body was falling apart. When I heard 'IV,' I thought, okay, now I'm going to be an invalid in the hospital for the next month. It's all over. Boy, what an education I got!" Jack not only had the nurse check his catheter and dressings at the office, he was able to go on business trips and have a nurse from the destination city continue his care.

Emily, a sixty-year-old dairy farmer born and raised in Wisconsin, had slowed some of her activities because of Lyme, but was relieved to find out that she didn't have to stay in the hospital for IV treatments. Twice a day she sat down, hooked up her medication, and read, knitted, or watched television until the forty-five minutes needed for the infusion were up. "Then I hit the barn again."

And Barbara, who despite her Lyme struggled to stay in school, would meet the home care nurse in the school nurse's office. In this way, she was able to keep up with her classes and get the critical supervision she needed.

There is a home health care boom going on with little sign of letting up. In 2000, Americans shelled out approximately $125 billion for nursing home and home health care services. And although this service is extremely convenient, it places the Lyme patient in an unusual position. After making it through the maze of doctors, tests, increasing symptoms, and finally diagnosis, the patient must then become an employer in a field in which few have expert knowledge.

HOME CARE CONTROVERSIES

Newspaper headlines have appeared in Lyme-endemic areas blasting physicians for referring patients to companies in which they have a financial interest. The implications were that all Lyme doctors who recommend companies are either getting kickbacks or own part of the company.

In other headline stories, home care companies have been exposed as charging inflated prices for medication. Where two grams of Claforan, prescribed as one gram twice a day, may cost $170 through one company, another might charge up to $450 for the same two grams.

And some insurance companies and HMOs, as well as Medicare, have been reluctant to cover portions of—or any— therapies provided by home health care companies. They have charged that money-hungry doctors refer patients for IV therapy even when they don't need it because the health care companies give the doctors kickbacks for those referrals.

What is a patient to do when confronted with another confusing choice after having IV therapy prescribed? The smart medical consumer will ask questions, and a lot of them, right from the beginning.

TWO TYPES OF IV THERAPY

Depending upon the patient's age and stage of Lyme disease, lifestyle, and the accessibility of veins, the doctor will recommend that either a "peripheral catheter" or a "central line" be put into the patient's body for administering medication.

Peripheral catheters are usually inserted into a vein in the forearm, although individual circumstances may occasionally dictate another site. This insertion is easily performed in the doctor's office, and the catheter (often called a Pic Line, Streamline,

or Landmark) can remain in the patient's arm, barring complications, for anywhere from two to six weeks before it needs to
be removed or replaced. Medication is infused through the vein,
either by gravity (the traditional hanging bag) or through one of
several "IV push" methods, which can include portable contain-
ers or time-release pumps.

A central line catheter is implanted in the chest area by a surgeon, and the medication goes directly into a vein, which trans-
fers it directly into the heart. This central line, usually referred to
as an "implanted port," can remain in a patient for months before
needing replacement. The site for the medication infusion would
be in either the upper arm or the chest area, and infusion is
accomplished in the same ways described for the peripheral line.

Both types of lines are easily camouflaged by clothing and do
not cause discomfort to the patient if inserted properly. One primary restriction is that they should not become wet or be
immersed—this means no swimming and that care must be
taken when bathing. Following the initial insertion, done either
in the doctor's office or in an ambulatory surgery unit, the continuing monitoring and care of the IV line is then referred to a
home health care company.

When a physician prescribes IV therapy, he or she may make
a recommendation for a preferred home health care company.
The hardest thing to remember at this point is that you, as the
patient or advocate, have a choice. For many who have searched
for a diagnosis, the doctor who finally pinpoints Lyme disease
may seem to wear wings and a halo, and they may be earned.
But asking the right questions is part of your therapeutic
alliance, and a reputable doctor will be straightforward in giving
reasons for preferring a company and will encourage you to
make some telephone calls before coming to a decision.

AM I COVERED?

Prior to selecting a home health care company, you should begin
by contacting your insurance company to find out what it will

cover in terms of home care. Since there are some policies that do not cover home care at all, you must first make this determination. If you have established that your company *will* cover some portion of home therapy, the following questions should be asked:

1. What is my deductible for home health care?
2. Is IV therapy covered entirely if taken at home or must I be in the hospital for some portion of it?
3. What percentage of the therapy is paid by the insurance company and what do I have to pay?
4. Is there a maximum benefit for home IV therapy, after which the company will discontinue coverage? What is that amount?
5. Does the company have a "case management" policy once the client has amassed large bills? This may indicate reassessment of the medical situation with the possibility of reduced coverage.
6. What is the name of the person with whom you will be dealing?

Once you have established the insurance company's coverage, the first decision to be made is whether to go with a local, national, or international home health care company.

SELECTING THE COMPANY

When ten-year-old Billy was diagnosed as needing intravenous therapy for disseminated Lyme disease, his mother, Marsha, decided to go with a local company. She knew the director of nursing and, in fact, had worked with her on a fund-raiser at church. Dealing with this company was like having a neighbor watching over her son. This was a relationship that worked well.

Carl needed a company that could accommodate his business travel schedule. As Midwest sales manager for a large pharmaceutical firm, he sought out a home health care company that could continue his IV supervision on the road, if need be. This relationship also worked well.

Carol also traveled, but her business travel as a fashion representative included trips to London, Paris, Rome, and sometimes Hong Kong. In order for her to continue working while on IV therapy, she needed to find a company that could accommodate *her* schedule, since overseas travel was usually a little less flexible than domestic. She, too, found a company that could provide continuity despite her location.

There are thousands of home health care companies—and many more springing up on a monthly basis—so it may seem a daunting task to sift through the names and make a decision as to which one would be right for your particular situation. Your first consideration should be whether to go with a company that is local, one that has offices in other states, or one that can serve you not only locally or nationally but internationally as well.

All things being equal (and we will discuss accreditation, personnel training, and services below), if the Lyme patient is not likely to travel out of state during the treatment, a local company could be ideal, but you should take the time to interview, by telephone, a representative from both the local and the national with local offices. It ultimately comes down to the person with whom you will be dealing on a weekly basis.

Once you have chosen the type of company, you should check the organization's accreditation. As of this writing, the accreditations needed vary from state to state. One standard of excellence, however, is whether the home health care company is Joint Commission Accredited, or Home Caring Council Accredited. These are voluntary certifications that require stringent guidelines for training, service, and quality control.

After having ascertained the company accreditation, you should then begin with the critical questions.

ASKING THE RIGHT QUESTIONS

Reputable home health care companies should be judged in three basic areas: patient services, personnel, and quality control. These three areas can be further broken down. The following guidelines can be used when shopping for a company.

■ Patient Services

1. Do you have a twenty-four-hour-a-day emergency number? What is your response time?
Whether you choose a local, national, or international company, home health care is all about providing local service on demand. The larger companies should have a local office from which they dispense medications and personnel. Emergencies and concerns arise at all hours of the day and night, and a patient should be able to call the company and have a nurse visit at three A.M. if necessary—and do so cheerfully and competently. Most reputable companies will have someone at your front door within fifteen minutes to half an hour.

2. What materials do you provide for patient education?
After the first dose of medication, which should be given in the doctor's office, and the first instruction on how to administer the medication yourself, the company should provide the patient and advocate with educational materials. This should not only include a step-by-step chart of how to administer the medication, but a "what if" list of possible concerns, signs of problems, and possible solutions, including calling the nurse. Some companies provide their Lyme patients with professionally produced videos, while others provide booklets, charts, and notebooks.

3. Do you encourage patient participation?
This covers everything from patients feeling at ease in asking questions outside the normally assigned appointment to reassur-

ing patients as to where their responsibilities lie. This may be particularly important when a child needs infusion therapy.

Sometimes, when you have multiple family members down with Lyme, the medication schedules can get a little confusing, particularly if people are suffering from short-term memory loss. The responsible company will work with them on setting up the schedules and lists and checking the medications off daily, to make sure everyone has theirs.

4. Are your charges line charges or bundled?

Upon being interviewed, some companies may tell you that each dose of Claforan will cost you $125–$170. What you need to find out is whether this figure applies just to the medication (a line charge), with separate charges for the nurse visit, the equipment, and twenty-four-hour emergency service, or whether it includes all those services as well as the medication (a bundled charge). Make sure you are comparing apples and apples when shopping for a company.

5. Will IV therapy be provided at various sites at the patient's convenience?

One day, the patient may need to be met at work in a particular time slot, or at school, rather than at the "normal" home location. Make sure your company has this flexibility.

6. What kind of support services are available?

Well-established and reputable companies will either offer, or have access to, a variety of services such as nutritional counseling, research data on Lyme disease, insurance company liaisons, and personal assistance in such areas as grocery shopping, bill paying, and transportation. Of particular importance is the company's help in dealing with insurance companies, as its personnel will likely have more experience in dealing with therapy reimbursements than the clients.

Because insurance companies like managed care as a type of

service, you may have to precertify that you have Lyme disease before treatment begins and then follow up with documentation on your progress. The therapies provided by a home care company are less expensive than if a patient were confined to a hospital, but they aren't cheap, so working with the insurance company is crucial.

■ Personnel

7. Do you provide a uniform standard of procedures for your nurses?
There are many skilled and experienced nurses from many fine institutions that teach IV procedures in very different fashions. One of the aspects of therapy you are "buying" from a home health care company is consistency in quality care. The company should provide an orientation and standardized process not only for its nurses but also for those who answer the telephone, deliver the medications, and assist patients in any of the supportive services.

8. Do you have a specially trained pediatric IV nurse available?
This should be insisted upon when the patient is a child. Not all nurses who have been trained on IV therapy have experience dealing with children, and this is critical. The emotional overlay in the family is different when it is the child on IV therapy. The technical aspect of working with smaller veins is more challenging, and adolescents and teens, in particular, are very body-conscious. You need a nurse who is sympathetic, experienced, and skilled in dealing with all these issues. Insist upon it; it's part of what you are paying for.

9. What type of ongoing training or assessment do you provide your staff?
Home care is personal care, and *everyone* who comes in contact with the patient—from the person answering the telephone to the person who delivers the weekly supply of medication—should

be accessible, helpful, and kind. One can get a sense of the company's standards simply by calling and asking a few questions. The more reputable companies will invite you in for a tour; your questions will be answered patiently and completely. You should never feel as though you are imposing on them. Remember, *you* are the boss who is prospectively hiring *them,* and you should be treated as such.

Many times, particularly with older patients who are reluctant to ask questions or complain to a nurse, the delivery person becomes the front-line representative for the company. There should be a system of feedback so that a patient's concerns can be reported to the case nurse or supervisor.

10. Can we change nurses if a problem occurs?

Not every nurse-and-patient combination is made in personality heaven. Despite a high competency level, the chemistry may just be off. Or the patient may have a legitimate concern about the nurse's skill. In both of these situations, the patient should have the right to change nurses without any anxiety of reprisals or an implication of "snitching." After all, you would have few reservations over complaining about service at a restaurant. Why should you show your health any less respect?

11. Do you have pharmacists on staff? Where? May I speak with them about my medication?

Again, whether a company is local, international, or in between, home health care is a local service and a patient has a right to speak with the pharmacist in charge. Beware the companies that have only technicians, or a consulting pharmacist. This is your life you are putting in their hands, and you want assurance that your medications are correct, fresh, and given personal attention.

12. Where is the closest office to me?

Home health care is a local market; procedures that may work in New York may not satisfy a patient in rural Georgia or

Florida. Nurses, drivers, and pharmacists should be local and "on call," with backup available twenty-four hours a day.

13. Do you pay physicians for referrals?

While this varies from state to state, it is generally a law that any physician who has a financial interest in a health care company to which he is referring patients have a public announcement card placed in a very visible location in the office. By the same token, it is illegal and inappropriate to pay physicians for referrals. The question then arises, "Is the physician earning so much with a home care company that he has an incentive to send patients into therapy even when it's not necessary?" Patients should ask about a doctor's financial interest in the company before making decisions about it.

■ Quality Control

14. How large a supply of equipment is delivered at a time? If we run out of something, can it be replaced?

Reputable companies will not deliver more than a week's worth of equipment for IV therapy (bandages, tape, syringes, saline, heparin, etc.) at a time. In addition, each patient must be supplied with an anaphylaxis kit in case of allergic reaction.

The visiting nurse should do an equipment assessment at each visit, with a follow-up telephone call from the company. A patient shouldn't have to run out to the drugstore to pick up rolls of tape. The thing to remember is that once the equipment has been delivered to you, it cannot be returned and recycled. (At least it should not be!) Therefore, you want enough to make it through the week, but not so much that you are wasting money on excess supplies.

15. How do you track a patient's progress?

A number of companies use the "one chart" system, whereby each person has a chart that contains contributions from not only the case nurse but the physician, pharmacist, delivery person, and anyone taking telephone calls from the patient. In this way, each patient's information is organized and complete. Other companies, like Coram Health Care, also feel strongly that a home chart, with complete assessments, updates, and nurses' comments, should be left with the patient. In this way, if there is a substitution of the visiting health worker for any reason, all of the patient's history is available. And since the home health care worker will often be the first to notice changes of any type, full and accurate communication must be maintained at all times. It is important for you, the medical consumer, to know that your therapy is part of a coordinated effort.

16. How often does the company have contact with my doctor?
Again, this goes back to coordinated care and open communication. Home health care is a team effort to get the patient well, and the physician and home health care professionals must keep each other apprised of any changes in the patient's condition. An attentive home care nurse will inform the patient's doctor of any changes on a routine basis.

17. Does the agency write a personalized care plan for each patient?
This may be a foregone conclusion if the home care company is accredited by the two large voluntary commissions, but it's a good question to ask nonetheless.

Finally, as with anything else, the best recommendation is word of mouth from those who have been through the same experience. If you are confused over home health care companies, begin by asking your physician or by contacting members of your local Lyme support group to find out which companies might successfully offer those services that satisfy your individual needs.

17.
What's Insurance For?

The tag lines are so darn enticing: "Feel Secure," "A Business of Caring," "What Works for You?," and "Turning Promise into Practice," to name just a few. They give you that warm and fuzzy they're-going-to-take-care-of-me feeling, don't they? Unfortunately, as millions who have gone head-to-head with dozens of insurance companies have discovered, a more accurate tag line could be: "You Bet Your Life!"

Scientists can research their brains out, independent institutions can conduct all the double-blind studies they want, and knowledgeable physicians can utilize all of their board-certified skills to create an effective protocol based on experience, documentation, and individualized attention to a patient's condition . . . but if the insurance company covering that patient decides it doesn't want to spend any more money on treatment of a certain disease—that patient doesn't get the needed medicine, tests, or treatment. And, all too often, people—including Lyme-infected people—will deteriorate and die.

In any other arena, this would be called a criminal act of negligence or fraud. In the insurance industry today, it's simply called "doing business."

Ask Dr. Ken Liegner about the seven-year-old Connecticut girl who was refused treatment for the bite of a deer tick in that hyperendemic Lyme area. She and her parents went through the progression of Lyme hell and misdiagnosis for months before she was taken to a more knowledgeable physician who recognized that the child was in a late disseminated stage and was displaying severe neurological problems. Placed on intravenous antibiotic therapy, she showed gradual but marked improvement. Then the insurance company's physician reviewer, acting on company policy, denied further treatment. The child went into a state of continual seizures as the antibiotics left her system. One month later, she was dead.

Or ask Marvina Lodge of Florida, whose son was born with congenital Lyme problems and has gone nearly deaf because the insurance company refuses to pay for the antibiotic treatment he requires. Or ask Leslie Salmon, whose three children all contracted Lyme disease and whose insurance company denied treatment after the company policy of four weeks of antibiotics had expired. Despite a "two-foot pile" of documentation, despite several expert witnesses, and despite her husband being the local police chief and who had spent his life in community service and paying insurance premiums, Leslie's family was forced to seek federal aid and accept donations from a fund-raiser held by town employees in empathy with the family's plight and the children's deterioration.

More than 43.6 million Americans do not have health insurance, according to the Census Bureau's latest figures. This is the highest jump of uninsureds in our country's history; the equivalent of the cumulative populations of twenty-four states plus the District of Columbia, according to Ron Pollack, executive director of Families USA, a national citizens' advocacy and information organization. But even many of those 168 million Americans who *do* have health insurance are finding that their insurance is anything but a guarantee when it comes to covering the cost of an illness like Lyme disease. More than 76.1 million people presently enrolled in the once-enticing HMOs find that their coverage does not extend to doctors and treatments for various specified diseases, such as Lyme disease. And by the year 2005, up to 60 percent of all working and retired adults who purchased long-term-care insurance, labeled the fastest-growing type of insurance today with more than six million active policies sold, may find themselves "uncared for" if their health problems are due to

Lyme. Reforming the health care system will require more than good intentions, money, and a decade of untangling the web of political ties that bind insurers to big business.

Currently, the guidelines of some of the nation's largest carriers will not allow for re-treatment or extended treatment of Lyme disease, and the initial treatment period is deemed to be twenty-eight days. This is in spite of documentation from around the country that a significant percentage of patients are outside of the "early treatment" parameters due to late diagnosis and the pathology of the organism itself.

In testifying before the New York State Assembly Committee on Health in November of 2001, Dr. Liegner, who has been a tireless advocate for Lyme patients everywhere, pleaded, "It is vital that treating physicians be enabled to exercise their individual clinical judgment as to choice and method of administration of antimicrobial agents and duration of treatment unencumbered by third party interference." Attempting to put the controversy and debate in perspective, he likened the official attitude toward Lyme disease to another spirochetal illness, syphilis. "There was bitter controversy at the turn of the twentieth century over what constituted appropriate treatment, duration of treatment, and criteria for cure. It has taken medical science more than four hundred years to understand syphilis as a chronic, multisystem infectious disease that evolves over time. We are but twenty-five years into understanding the spirochetal infection known as Lyme disease."

Like Lyme disease, syphilis patients can test negative, display progressive neurological impairment, and be affected by both prior antibiotic treatment and tired immune systems. The major difference between the research development and treatment for syphilis and Lyme disease is the injection of the insurance industry into the diagnosis and treatment of ill people. "Since Metropolitan Life Insurance Company had an integral formative role in the formation of the National Institutes of Health during the 1920s, this raises the issue of possible ongoing undue influence of the insurance industry in setting national public health priorities," said Liegner.

Despite international and domestic research to the contrary, despite the CDC's emphatic statements that Lyme disease is a clinical diagnosis, that chronic Lyme disease is a serious condition and should be treated appropriately, and that CDC criteria for tracking Lyme disease should not be used for any other purpose, most insurance companies have glommed onto CDC restrictive criteria as well as a set of medical practice guidelines concerning Lyme disease issued by the Infectious Diseases Society of America (IDSA). These guidelines assert that there is "no significant evidence that chronic Lyme disease exists" and that there "is no role for treatment with antibiotics beyond one or at most two months for any case of Lyme disease."

"Physicians whose prescribing patterns do not conform to IDSA guidelines have been targeted and reported to state departments of health for investigation for medical misconduct," Liegner told the New York State Assembly. "It is a 'no lose' proposition for the insurance industry. This enmeshes such physicians in a costly, stressful, and time-consuming administrative process that pits them individually against the vast power and resources of the State and jeopardizes their practices, professional reputations, and financial solvency. Even if they win, they lose. Not surprisingly, persons with chronic Lyme are having increasing difficulty finding any physician anywhere willing to see them.

"At the very least, the IDSA guidelines are highly scientifically biased. At worst, they may be frankly fraudulent," said Liegner. "The document omits scores of articles from the worldwide peer-reviewed literature demonstrating the reality of chronic persistent infection despite prior antibiotic treatment. No clinicians who actually care for Lyme disease patients were invited to participate in drafting the guidelines and the sole academician in the IDSA, known to acknowledge the existence of chronic Lyme, was purged from the committee drafting the document. The single greatest obstacle to badly needed progress in development of improved methods of diagnosis and treatment for Lyme disease is the chronic persistent denial of chronic persistent infection in the illness. Such denial, in the face of so much objective evidence to the contrary, must be viewed as a type of social pathology."

This concern over insurance carriers and their physicians ignoring the reality of the disease and supportive documentation motivated U.S. Public Law 107-116, which was signed by President George W. Bush on January 10, 2002, under the auspices of the Departments of Labor, Health and Human Services Appropriations Act. A portion of it reads:

> The Committee is distressed in hearing of the widespread misuse of the current Lyme disease surveillance case definition. While the CDC does state that "this surveillance case definition was developed for national reporting of Lyme disease, it is NOT appropriate for clinical diagnosis," the definition is reportedly misused as a standard of care for health care reimbursement, (test) product development, medical licensing hearings, and other legal cases. The CDC is encouraged to aggressively pursue and correct the misuse of this definition. This includes issuing an alert to the public and physicians, as well as actively issuing letters to places misusing this definition.

While this sounds amazingly supportive, the harsh realities of insurance coverage have increasingly put Lyme patients in the no-win situation whereby one company declares them well and therefore ineligible for continued coverage, yet another company labels them as having a preexisting condition if they attempt to apply for new insurance.

In addition, because states are prohibited from regulating self-insured employers under the Employee Retirement Income and Security Act (ERISA), employees' coverage can be pulled at any time, and smaller insurance companies have the option of canceling policies of the sickest patients in order to save money. This was evident when the state of California gave permission to the Great Republic Insurance Company to cancel fourteen thousand policies overnight, including those of a woman who had just learned she had cancer and a man scheduled for heart surgery.

Many insurance companies, utilizing the medical profession's own competing factions and polarity regarding Lyme disease, maintain that treatment beyond thirty days is experimental and noncurative. Clinicians and patients, pointing to continuing published research discoveries and the individual's own response to therapy, angrily charge that insurance companies are not fulfilling their contractual obligations, are practicing medicine without a license, and are forcing policyholders and their children into chronic ill health and financial ruin when the client finally attempts to collect on paid-up policies.

There are insurance companies with integrity across the country that *are* covering their policyholders who contract Lyme. Unfortunately, these are too few and far between—but they have earned the undying loyalty of their clients. The fear of losing coverage is so great among Lyme patients, however, that in interviewing people across the country, I was repeatedly begged *not* to mention the names of these reputable carriers because their clients are terrified that their companies will join the bandwagon of dumping Lyme patients.

The major insurers have traditionally had the credibility of institutional status and billions of dollars of assets in their arsenal of weapons against a policyholder's claim. Yet thousands of sick Davids are developing new weapons and are increasingly taking on the Goliaths of the insurance industries, with mixed results. Major lawsuits in the worker's compensation arena have been won when Lyme was proven to be contracted on the job, and many insurance industry giants have been directed by the courts to continue covering IV treatments.

THE INSURANCE EDGE

People buy insurance as protection against and compensation for adversity. The concept, as it originated, seems simple enough. Mr. X pays Company A ten dollars a week for health coverage.

When Mr. X gets sick, the company is expected to pay the bills less whatever deductible is agreed upon, as set forth in the original agreement. Whether Company A makes or loses money along the way is generally immaterial to Mr. X, as long as he receives the medicine and treatment he has paid for when he needs it.

As the theory progressed to industry status and simple policies mutated into a cornucopia of variables, insurance companies, now inflated with investments, landholdings, personnel, and self-importance, began changing the rules of the original game when faced with situations that affected the bottom line. This is all the more upsetting to the American public because it views the insurance industry not merely as a business but as a caretaker of health and welfare. After all, these companies are influencing the course—and sometimes the end—of people's lives.

This pluralistic view finds little sympathy for an industry that avows allegiance first to its shareholders, and second to its policyholders. Representatives complain that the public wants more and unlimited coverage for less money so the insurance industry has developed several new programs—called "consumer-driven care"—whereby policyholders are given a choice of lower rates and coverage in exchange for betting that they will stay healthy. The public complains that it has paid high premiums for years (health insurance costs constitute more than 20 percent of the Detroit automakers' total wage bill, for example), only to be cut off when needs arise. And according to Hewitt Associates, an international human resources consulting firm based in Illinois, and Mercer Human Resource Consulting, which surveyed more than 3,000 employers representing 90 million employees nationwide, HMO rates are rising another 17.7 percent on average and overall insurance costs are going up another 14 percent in 2004.

Collectively, Blue Cross and Blue Shield companies probably represent the largest health insurance carrier in the country. Approximately half of the Blue Cross claims by Lyme patients applying for extended treatment have been denied. Other giants such as Prudential, Aetna, Cigna, and Oxford also uphold the "four weeks of therapy is sufficient" treatment for Lyme disease.

Dr. Stanley Harris trained as a pediatrician and worked his way up through the medical hierarchy, managing eleven acute care hospitals and multiple health centers in the New York City system before attaining the position of senior medical director for Horizon Blue Cross Blue Shield of New Jersey. His state is the fourth highest in the nation in Lyme disease claims, only slightly behind Rhode Island, New York, and Connecticut. Despite the fact that he has attended Lyme disease conferences and met with clinicians who treat multitudes of patients, he says that the policy of the company to stick to the thirty-day coverage is based on published literature and admittedly conservative teaching centers, but that there is a recognized potential for bias.

But even within a conglomerate like Blue Cross Blue Shield, differences in practice exist. Tad Dadisman, director of preventive medicine for the Washington, D.C.–based CareFirst Blue Cross Blue Shield, which services 3.2 million in the mid-Atlantic region, says, "Chronic Lyme disease is a real entity and it's difficult to diagnose correctly, so treatment can be somewhat empirical. We don't get in the way of practitioners' treating their folks for something like this."

Another weapon in the arsenal of insurance company claims offices is the bureaucratic tap dance done on appeals of company policy.

Kevin, his wife, and his daughter all contracted Lyme disease while on a family vaction in the Southwest. Since it affected each differently, taking varied times to disseminate and become debilitating, they were each in varied disseminated late stages before the disease was diagnosed and treatment begun. Four weeks into the treatment, their insurance company discontinued coverage. All three family members began sliding backward when treatment was stopped. Kevin's twelve-year-old daughter began having tremors and heart palpitations, which landed her in the hospital. They began the process of appealing the insurance company decision.

While Kevin filled out the necessary appeal forms and waited, he took out a second mortgage on his house and depleted his savings in an attempt to pay for continued IV therapy. Weeks passed, during which the company said it had misplaced the file, please file again; the caseworker was on vacation; the file had to go to the home office; the file had to go to medical consultants; the caseworker quit and a new caseworker needed time to acclimate; the file was misplaced, would he please file again?

At the end of nine weeks, and still with no response from the insurance company, Kevin had to give up his own treatment so he could continue to pay for his family's. At the end of eleven weeks, his wife gave up her treatment so their daughter could continue to fight Lyme.

Today Kevin is in litigation with his insurer. He is in a wheelchair; his wife uses a cane. Their daughter is off IV therapy and on oral antibiotics but is suffering from depression and guilt, feeling she is to blame for her parents' debilitated condition.

As one West Coast physician, who has counseled numerous patients on fighting for their paid coverage, says, "We send the charts, the charts get lost. We recopy them. The company changes personnel. I would have to stop practicing medicine and just spend my days helping patients fight the insurance companies if they were to be successful. That's what the companies count on; they know we don't have that kind of time and the patients are often too sick to follow through. The vicious circle is that, if they don't follow through, they get even sicker. Either way, the patient loses."

This underscores the need for a patient advocate, as it would become the advocate's responsibility to assist the ill person in petitioning for continued coverage. On a more formal basis, Lyme patients across the country may have found representation through independent organizations formed to do battle with the insurance industry.

PATIENTS FIND A VOICE

People in Donna's old neighborhood called her family "the Lymies," but Donna, facing financial devastation, isn't laughing.

The forty-four-year-old nurse and her three daughters are all victims of Lyme disease. Tina, fifteen, and Ceil, thirteen, have been on intravenous treatment intermittently for two years. Tina, who suffers from severe eye pain and loss of peripheral vision and has difficulty concentrating, is unable to attend school regularly and studies at home with a tutor's help.

Ceil, who is currently on intravenous treatment, goes to school part-time. She, too, has headaches, joint pain, neurologic impairment, dizziness, and fatigue.

Karen, the eight-year-old, displayed few symptoms until she began having episodes of tremors. Then the joint pain, stomach cramps, headaches, and heart palpitations kicked in.

Prudential Insurance informed Donna that she and her daughters should be well, that further treatment was deemed not medically reasonable by the company, and that further medications and services for Lyme disease would not be covered.

Donna, a single parent, is particularly upset because she had been buying medical supplies directly from the hospital and administering the medication herself, rather than paying a home health care company. Despite the savings, she has been forced to sell her home and borrow from relatives in order to meet the cost of medical treatment. Not only is she upset, she is angry. "I am outraged to be told by an insurance company that, according to their textbooks, we are supposed to be well, so they aren't paying for our medical treatment. Is this why I have contributed to their company for all these years? Since when did insurance companies get medical degrees?"

Donna's outrage has been matched by a number of legislators primarily from the Northeast, spurred by their own family experiences with Lyme and Lyme activists. Connecticut State Attorney General Richard Blumenthal has made no secret of his intent to pressure insurance companies to live up to the spirit and letter of their commitments to the citizens of the state. Despite being criticized by many captains of industry as politically suicidal in a state where the biggest source of revenue is the insurance industry, Blumenthal's passionate watchdog tactics regarding health, the environment, and children's issues resulted in his reelection in 2002 to an unprecedented fourth term. A resident of Greenwich and father of four children, Blumenthal worked for and applauded the U.S. Supreme Court's recent decision affirming the rights of patients to an external review of HMO decisions and forcing HMOs to pay if the review determines additional care is warranted.

"This decision is a solid step supporting state protection of patient rights, but more needs to be done to secure health care rights of citizens," says Blumenthal. "My hope is that the ruling will provide momentum and lead to both state and federal measures enhancing protection against HMO abuses, and we will vigorously pursue pending cases." This isn't just talk from a man who filed lawsuits in 2003 against seven of the largest pharmaceutical firms in the country—including Schering-Plough, Aventis, GlaxoSmithKline, and Pharmacia Corporation—for inflating their prices on drugs for cancer, respiratory illnesses, and other serious diseases. In addition, after launching an investigation into an Aetna/U.S. Healthcare contract that would require physicians to sign a document imposing restrictions on their care of a patient, Attorney General Blumenthal called for legislation clarifying health care fraud that would give his office greater latitude in pursuing individual cases. "I'm very concerned that doctors are being pressured to give patients less care and inadequate care as a result of abusive and coercive contract provisions," he said. "The corporate bottom line shouldn't undercut the quality of medical care. The result may be cutting health care corners to cut costs and so imperiling lives."

After Connecticut, Rhode Island has the highest rate of reported Lyme infection, with an estimated 81.3 out of 100,000 people infected in 2002 alone. The numbers are still rising, says Dr. Patricia Nolan, director of the Rhode Island Department of Health. Using extremely conservative numbers, this meant that the state would be experiencing an economic drain of at least $30 million a year just due to Lyme disease. Governor Lincoln

Almond formed the Commission on Lyme and Other Tick-Borne Illnesses in 2001 and for a year held public hearings on the problem. Rhode Island legislators listened to Lyme victims who had become financially destitute when their insurance companies refused to pay for doctor-ordered tests and medications, to others who had lost family members to the disease because of their inability to pay out of pocket for antibiotics, and to researchers and physicians representing a wide range of opinions.

As a result of those hearings and supporting research, current Governor Donald Carcieri signed into law the Lyme Disease Diagnosis and Treatment Act, which, sponsored by Senator Michael Damiani, and Representative Raymond Gallison, passed in both the Rhode Island House and Senate on July 2, 2003. According to the act, chronic Lyme disease is an entity that requires long-term antibiotic care and this long-term treatment must be covered by state-licensed insurance companies beginning in 2004. The act also protects physicians from censure simply because they are treating Lyme patients long term. "This is a patient bill, not a vested interest bill," said Pat Smith, president of the LDA. The 2003 report on the Rhode Island Governor's Commission on Lyme and Other Tick-Borne Illnesses also outlines a plan to protect the health of the general population (discussed in chapter 20).

On a federal level, Senator Christopher Dodd (D-Conn.) and Senator Rick Santorum (R-Penn.) instigated the Lyme Disease Initiative, which allocated $125 million over five years for research on all aspects of Lyme and requested that the General Accounting Office investigate allegations of the misspent federal funds targeted for Lyme disease research.

Equitable treatment from insurance companies is also the province of Families USA, located in Washington, D.C. Formerly the Villers Foundation, it was founded in 1981 by Philippe Villers and his wife, Kate, to reform the health care system in the United States so that it assures universal access to care. Villers, who fled to the United States when he was five years old to escape Nazi persecution, grew up to become the creator of

Computervision, a successful computer company. The foundation is his contribution to his adopted country. It provides grants and advocacy for those seeking redress in the health care arena. Under its Health Assistance Partnership, Families USA assistance to consumers ranges from education and mediating solutions to investigating complaints and actually representing consumers in hearings. (See appendix C for contact information.)

One New Jersey internist who treats hundreds of Lyme patients has been prodding newspapers, institutions, and legislators with facts regarding the need for long-term treatment in cases of disseminated Lyme. Armed with both clinical experience and published research, he scoffs at what he terms the "Bermuda Triangle logic" of those companies denying their Lyme patient policyholders treatment coverage.

"In a letter to a patient of mine, an insurance company wrote: 'There seems to be no documentation that the patient did in fact have Lyme disease' and 'there is no documentation of central nervous system Lyme disease.' This patient [who had been diagnosed with Lyme on the recommended clinical basis] had severe cognitive impairment demonstrated on neuropsychiatric examination by an independent clinician," said the doctor. "He also had many of the cognitive problems that can be resolved using prolonged IV and oral antibiotic treatment. The patient, now on pulse therapy, continues to improve." If some parts of the medical community still say this type of successful long-term treatment isn't sufficient "clinical proof," then many other accepted treatments now used successfully aren't justified either. These include the prescribing of Inderal for migraine headaches and nitroglycerin for treating chest pain.

Insurance company consultants have not been able to prove that twenty-eight days of treatment for Lyme is curative. On the contrary, abbreviated therapy in many patients permits survival of the Lyme disease spirochete and fails to provide enduring symptom relief. This has been established through meticulous documentation and multiple research studies worldwide. Often, symptoms return within one to two months after a short course of antibiotics. Dr. Burrascano and others have reported that patients had progressive relief and fewer relapses with longer antibiotic treatment, whether IV or oral. I feel the insurance companies have adopted an inappropriate standard of care which is inconsistent with the available research and patient experience.

The insurance industry's stated policy of not covering treatment beyond thirty days because such treatment is not curative and is "therefore experimental" doesn't hold water when one looks at its coverage of other diseases that—unlike Lyme disease—do not have a definitive cause or endpoint. Illnesses such as fibromyalgia, chronic fatigue syndrome, chronic mono, or even multiple sclerosis have stumped the researchers for years and their sufferers number in the millions. Yet for as long as symptoms are present, treatment is covered.

The bottom-line decision by insurance companies not to cover Lyme patients beyond a limited time is a financial one.

Since the positive aspect of low medical costs through HMOs is derived from strict cost-containment practices and case managers who are paid to deny claims, and thereby save the company money, Lyme disease, with its potentially expensive and long treatment schedule, presents a major problem.

Chicago attorney Judee Gallagher, former counsel to the Illinois State Medical Society's Office of Contractual Services, has been repeatedly called upon to give advice regarding insurance and HMO coverage and liabilities. In an article for *Physician's Management,* she referred to the fact that, increasingly, HMOs are being cited as defendants in malpractice cases but have averted unfavorable verdicts if they can show that the physicians involved agreed in advance that the HMOs' cost-containment actions and payment denials would not affect medical care.

Clinicians who are knowledgeable regarding Lyme disease would most likely not agree to such absolute payment restrictions, which would also restrict effective medical care, so, once again, the onus is on the medical consumer to beware.

MAKING YOUR INSURANCE PAY

While I was updating this book, I received a communication from my own Aetna HMO informing me that from here on out, certain medications that are prescribed by physicians must first be approved by Aetna before I can expect to have the cost covered. Further, the physician involved must call Aetna and get authorization for the drug. "If the request is approved, your physician will be notified and the drug will then be covered," says this communication. "For instance, some drugs are more likely than others to be taken incorrectly. Sometimes they may be prescribed for inappropriate reasons or used in amounts that exceed recommendations for dosage or length of treatment." It sounds as though Aetna, like many other companies, is launching yet another creatively aggressive attack aimed at restricting physicians from practicing the medicine they were trained to practice.

Prophylactically, the best advice is to be sure you understand your health insurance policy and to review it periodically as family situations change. Most of us get those policy booklets and throw them into a file cabinet or drawer until we are in a desperate or litigious situation. Review the following:

- How much is your deductible? Is it per illness, per person, per year, or per family?
- What benefits are specifically covered? Look for mention of home care.
- What benefits are excluded? Generally, anything not specifically mentioned as a benefit is excluded.
- What is the lifetime maximum the plan will pay? What is the maximum it will pay for each illness?
- Under what conditions can the insurer cancel your plan?
- Are there limits on the types of services that are of interest to you? What are the limits on preexisting conditions?

If you have been diagnosed with disseminated Lyme and your physician recommends continued treatment but your insurance company refuses to continue coverage, the best advice given by the experts is "Don't give up!" Here are the key elements in fighting for insurance coverage:

▪ Document everything! This includes any communications via phone, fax, or e-mail with your physician, your child's teachers, your employer, or any other supportive official. Of major assistance is the journal that I recommended you keep (see chapter 4). Continued documentation of the illness, symptoms, treatment, and reactions to treatment provides you with supporting evidence with which to fight.

▪ Protest vigorously, using all available procedures dictated by both your insurance company and your state. Exhaust all your options under your contract and make copies of everything in case your file "gets misplaced." Contact your state and federal representatives for assistance. Make sure you include a "bulleted" sheet of the basic facts of your case, including contact information on the insurance company, your employer, and yourself.

▪ If appealing an insurance company decision, stay on top of it. Do not let weeks pass before following up on the course of your case. Continue to document your actions, the people you spoke with at the company, and the elapsed time involved, in addition to any reactions to stopping medication, if that becomes financially necessary. Ask your physician to send a strongly worded letter to the company stating that its action/inaction is impacting on the health of the patient. This may get the attention of the medical director, bypassing the clerical personnel who are handling routine claims.

▪ Appeal directly to the state if you have exhausted your insurance company appeal system. This is an option that few seem aware of, according to a recent Kaiser Family Foundation survey. In response to the problems many consumers have had with managed care, a number of states now allow external appeals. These include: Arizona, California, Colorado, Connecticut, Delaware, Florida, Georgia, Hawaii, Illinois, Indiana, Iowa, Kansas, Louisiana, Maryland, Michigan, Minnesota, Missouri, Montana, New Hampshire, New Jersey, New Mexico, New York,

Ohio, Oklahoma, Pennsylvania, Rhode Island, Tennessee, Texas, Utah, Vermont, Virginia, and Washington. There is usually a specified time frame to be followed, so call your state's insurance commission and find out exactly what documentation you must submit.

■ Check out the website www.NeedyMeds.com, a registered non-profit in Pennsylvania that was founded by a social worker and a physician. The site is an information source where you can learn about patient-assistance programs for those who cannot afford their medications. NOTE: They cannot help you with your individual problems, only provide information with which to help yourself.

■ Ask your physician to contact the pharmaceutical maker of the antibiotic you need and request a form for indigent benefits. A number of companies do provide medicine at a lower rate if the patient qualifies financially. You must do the legwork, however, working in concert with your physician.

■ Become politically active through a support group or by contacting your state legislators and holding them accountable. Remember, you may be sick, but those elected officials *work for you*. Give them a job to do!

■ Do not give up—you are not alone. If necessary, seek the outside support (this includes the media) of those who have experience in fighting for insurance claims and make your voice heard. Our political structure is such that you will be more successful if you can demonstrate support in numbers, and this will, in turn, provide your legislators with credibility to press your demands among their colleagues.

The injustice against Lyme patients by some members of the insurance industry is not going to be "cured" by anyone *but* Lyme patients and their advocates. The fight must be continued on a higher plane if families who are already struggling on so many fronts are to be able to enjoy paid treatment until they are well.

18.

Diet and Nutrition

Everyone is an expert these days on what you should and shouldn't eat. It seems as though each week brings another fad diet backed by its own coterie of celebrity fans. But "diet" is not necessarily synonymous with "nutrition," and when your body is ill, when it has been invaded by a spirochete that is determined to beat down your immune system and overtake your everyday life, taking antibiotics isn't going to do the total job of getting you well again.

So it should come as little surprise that those in the throes of Lyme disease can also take a proactive stance in reboosting the immune system and revitalizing the body. And yes, although it is difficult to believe, you *can* overcome Lyme's insidious effects and regain your health. But it takes active involvement on the patient's part, not complacent reliance on the treating physician or the antibiotics, whose only purpose is to destroy the spirochete.

Before we proceed to the nutritional rehabilitation of the body, there is one essential caveat the Lyme patient must remember. In order for any Lyme therapy to be successful, the patient must take the right medications in the manner prescribed, give up alcohol and tobacco, and get a daily dose of rest.

Of course, there are some who are going to shake their heads at this point and say, "Hey, no problem with taking the medicine, but . . . *smoking*? I can't give up smoking during this stressful time. And how can I live without my glass of wine with dinner?"

The harsh reality is that, if you truly want to get well, abstinence is part of the protocol. Instead of throwing up more obstacles to your recovery, by abstaining from tobacco, drugs, and alcohol, you'll give your body a fighting chance against Lyme.

Dr. Joseph Territo is the quintessential family doctor. In practice for over thirty years, he not only commands a loyal following of multigenerational patients, but also hosts radio talk shows in both New York and Rhode Island on the subject of living well naturally. Because he is located in Lyme-endemic New Jersey, Lyme patients have infiltrated his practice. He treats them with a combination of old-fashioned good sense, antibiotics, and a complete regimen of nutritional supplements.

"The protocol for Lyme disease *must* be individualized," he says. "Facts such as symptoms, approximate duration of infection, age of the patient, and previous medical history must all be taken into consideration. This means spending time with the patient, particularly on the first visit."

Territo has had remarkable success in getting his Lyme patients over the hump of lingering symptoms by using a rigorous nutritional program that includes:

1. A low-fat menu
2. An abundance of fresh or frozen vegetables
3. Avoidance of caffeine (that's right, no alcohol, no cigarettes, and no high-test java either!)
4. Avoidance of yeast-containing products
5. Adequate vitamin supplements
6. Avoidance of chocolate, aged cheese, and broccoli for headache-prone patients

"Although I am a great advocate of the use of vitamins and supplements, nothing can replace a good, well-balanced menu," says Territo. "Unfortunately, with prolonged antibiotic therapy, changes can take place in the lining of the intestine that must be combated."

These changes include the destruction of "friendly" bacteria, resulting in candida, or yeast infections; a pseudo-colitis, the so-called leaky-gut syndrome; and reduced absorption through the lining of the membrane. Any of these can be caused by long-term antibiotic therapy and can be addressed through over-the-counter supplements easily obtainable from your local health food store.

Traditionally, medical schools have not taught nutrition and preventive medicine to its students, but many physicians—particularly Lyme-literate doctors—understand the value of building up the wonderful machine that is the body while relieving painful symptoms through nutritional supplements. The list of suggested supplements that follows was gleaned from the recommendations of several knowledgeable doctors who insist that their Lyme patients incorporate good nutritional habits into their daily routines in order to boost the immune system, combat varied Lyme symptoms, and rebuild muscles.

1. A good, all-purpose multivitamin with minerals, such as MV-75 or Life Pack multivitamins that target specific genders, age groups, and problems.

2. Acidophilus—essential to maintain the normal balance of flora in the bowels and gastrointestinal tract, particularly for anyone on high doses of antibiotics (more on this later).

3. Vitamin C—1,000 mg twice a day if patient can tolerate it. Not only does vitamin C play an important role in free radical protection, but it also helps to boost immunity and assist in fighting inflammation.

4. Magnesium—1 tablet twice a day helps counteract twitches, muscle spasms, cramps, and general weakness. It may also help increase your energy level and restore cognitive abilities. This should be a part of everyone's dietary routine but is particularly important for Lyme patients.

5. Beta-carotene—25 mg twice a day. This powerful antioxidant has earned its reputation for protecting your body from damaging free radicals as well as helping to boost immunity and improve eyesight.

6. Coenzyme Q-10—a vitamin B–like compound that the body produces naturally when it is well and functioning; should be taken until infection is controlled. Heart biopsy studies of Lyme patients

indicate that they should take between 200 and 300 mg daily of the standard CoQ-10 or 90 mg of the well-absorbed, highly purified cystalline CoQ-10 sold by Pharmanex.

7. Echinacea—an over-the-counter vitamin supplement shown to be helpful in fighting chronic viral illnesses. The liquid form contains alcohol and should be avoided. This supplement is best utilized when "pulsed" for two to three weeks on and then one week off, since its benefits wear off with constant use.

8. BioGinkgo—a pharmaceutical-grade product recommended by Dr. Joe Burrascano and available from Pharmanex. Ginkgo biloba has been shown to increase blood flow to the brain and other parts of the body. Patient reports indicate clearer thinking and improved memory functions, though Burrascano warns that you should begin with a low dosage, then slowly increase, since a pressure-type vascular headache can result from the sudden increased circulation.

9. Milk thistle—175 mg three times daily to support liver function.

10. Essential fatty acids—result in a vast improvement in memory and concentration, a lessening of fatigue, aches, vertigo, and dizziness, and an alleviation of depression. Can be found as plant oils, which include evening primrose oil, black currant seed or borage oil, and fish oils that contain omega-3.

CANDIDA

Candida—or yeast infection—is not a uniquely feminine condition. People of any age and gender who take megadoses of antibiotics for a prolonged period of time (beyond two weeks), can develop yeast infections, and they *can* be sexually transmitted.

In the natural state of affairs, our gastrointestinal tract is home to many varieties of organisms, some friendly, some not so friendly. The friendly bacteria maintain a normal ecological balance in the intestines by suppression of yeast growth and other detrimental organisms. When antibiotics are taken for an extended period, an upset in the balance of GI tract promotes the growth of yeast, a single-cell organism that has the capability of rapid, uncontrolled multiplication. In other words, it can hit you like a ton of bricks!

While the media would have you believe that only women contract yeast infections in their genitals, and a quick heart-to-heart on the beach with a close friend will point you in the right direction, the real story is a little more complicated.

Yeast infections—a common side effect of Lyme disease because of the antibiotic treatment—can affect the skin and cause excessive perspiration, as well as flatulence, abdominal distress, headaches, fatigue, painfully swollen and irritated genitals in both sexes, joint pain, and leakage of toxins from the intestines into the circulatory system.

While eating yogurt is beneficial and should be part of one's daily diet, taking tablets of pure acidophilus—the same lactobacillus found in a less-concentrated form in yogurt—is even more advantageous to one's health because it replenishes the intestinal flora and reduces the risk and/or effect of yeast infections.

I've spoken with Lyme patients who have complained that they eat a cup of yogurt and take one acidophilus tablet each day and they *still* have yeast problems. There are two reasons for this. The first is that they are not taking *enough* acidophilus. When my son was ill, it was recommended that he take a *handful* of acidophilus tablets each day, and he consequently had very little difficulty with yeast. Secondly, the candida might be systemic. If this is the case, then, in addition to the acidophilus, your physician might prescribe Diflucan or Nizoral for two weeks at full dose, then a reduced dosage for maintenance therapy.

A multimodal attack on the spirochete that causes Lyme disease has proven to be the most effective way for a patient to regain his or her good health. While special attention to diet and nutrition are essential, there are several other adjunctive therapies that have proven successful (see chapter 19)—and a few of which you must beware.

COLLOIDAL SILVER, PYGNOGENOL, AND CORAL CALCIUM SUPREME

One supplement that has captured the attention of Lyme sufferers and stirred up a controversy is colloidal silver. Colloidal silver is simply a mixture of minute silver metal particles in a liquid base bottled for consumption. It has been considered a treatment for bacterial, viral, and fungal infections since the 1800s. Before the advent of modern antibiotics, doctors used many of the silver preparations on the market to treat everything from sore throats to warts.

Colloidal silver again made the news during the SARS outbreak when manufacturers claimed that it would prevent the SARS virus from entering the body. An investigation by *Consumer Reports,* however, debunked that assertion: "There's certainly no data that have shown silver to prevent viruses from invading your body," said Irwin Berlin, M.D., chief of pulmonary critical care at Elmhurst Hospital Center in Queens, New York, and an expert on SARS. Although silver may have mild antiseptic powers, it's too weak to be effective against most bacteria or viruses.

Colloidal silver is approved by the Food and Drug Administration, but is classified as a supplement rather than a drug. That is both good and bad news. Since the FDA does not regulate these supplements, they are easy to obtain. By the same token, manufacturers do not have to provide any proof of safety or efficacy. No blind studies have been done; no controlled analyses have been made.

Silver is an essential trace element required by our bodies in minute amounts. Most of what we take in from our diet, however, is ionic rather than metallic. Manufacturers and advocates tout colloidal silver as a natural antibiotic, an immune system booster, and a natural healing property that can relieve pain and suppress the Lyme spirochete. There seems to be little doubt that some people feel much better while taking colloidal silver, but there are also a number who have experienced such side effects as graying of the skin and eyeballs, and fingernails turning bluish. In addition, there have been complaints regarding neuro-logical impairment. This is *not* something Lyme sufferers need to add to their chest of woes.

Lyme patients should exercise common sense in using colloidal silver until solid research, rather than just anecdotal testimony, supports both the amount necessary to be effective and its efficacy in treating Lyme disease.

Pygnogenol, often paired with colloidal silver as the "dynamic duo" of Lyme relief, is a powerful antioxidant gleaned from the bark of pine trees in France. Antioxidants have long been accepted as aids in fighting the free radicals floating through our systems. As in the case of colloidal silver, pygnogenol should be viewed as an adjunctive supplement to a healthful diet, rather than a cure in and of itself.

Another supplement that many Lyme sufferers have been looking into is something called Coral Calcium Supreme, the subject of infomercials running on four major cable networks. According to the manufacturers, this product—gleaned from dead marine coral off the coast of Japan—can relieve the symptoms of everything from MS to heart disease and cancer. With so many women, in particular, conscious of bone density and the need for calcium even during the best of times, many have invested in what they perceive to be a "super calcium." It is important to know that in June of 2003, after an investigation into manufacturers' claims, the Federal Trade Commission filed charges against the manufacturers of Coral Calcium Supreme for fraudulent advertising.

An argument rages on, but the point is, even with dietary supplements, you must put on your medical consumer's cap and do your homework.

In addition to nutritional supplements to help get your body back to good health, a number of adjunctive therapies have been found useful by many Lyme sufferers and their physicians. Although a few of these are just downright dangerous.

19.

Adjunctive and Supportive Therapies

The doctor of the future will give no medicine but will inter-est his patients in the care of the human frame, in diet, and in the cause and prevention of disease.

—Thomas A. Edison

Gerald had been on antibiotics for Lyme disease for fifteen months when his chiropractor placed him on a definitive program of aerobic exercise, nutritional supplements, and acupuncture therapy. Within six weeks, Gerald was finally off medication and feeling healthier than he had in more than two years.

In California, ads promising a Lyme cure through meditation were published in a number of periodicals. The meditation course cost Elise $150. She said the only difference it made in her life was that she was $150 poorer and ashamed at having been taken as a fool.

In one tiny Atlantic Seaboard town, a man who holds no major certifications sells a serum marketed for Lyme disease patients. Since the serum is not a drug and he makes no promises, he is untouched by the law. But respectable local practitioners of holistic therapies and traditional physicians continually have to warn patients away from this man.

In Texas, twelve-year-old Melissa thought she had died and gone to heaven when her mother told her she was going to begin HBO therapy for her Lyme disease. Melissa thought she was going to sit around and just watch television all day. She quickly found out that what she was going to do was be put in a hyperbaric oxygen chamber for an hour at a time.

Most people laugh when confronted with vignettes about snake oil salesmen trying to persuade an innocent audience that the product they hawk will relieve their heartburn, cure their warts, give them fresh breath, and enhance their sexual performance. Yet those same people, in the midst of a chronic, painful, and debilitating illness like Lyme disease, can fall for a modern version of the snake oil pitch that promises pain relief and revived good health. These victims and others in the United States will spend whatever it takes, but they are the ones who wind up "taken," to the tune of approximately $40 billion per year.

There *are* some legitimate supportive therapies available for the relief of Lyme disease symptoms, and I will discuss those shortly. They are designed to boost the body's own immune system, suppress the spirochete, or recapture the strength lost from extensive illness and antibiotic therapy. The trick is learning to distinguish them from the sham therapies that abound.

MEDICAL CONSUMER, BEWARE!

For most of us who are plunged into the world of Lyme disease, the whole medical arena is like a trip to Mars. We are suddenly learning a new lingo, dealing with alien professionals, and navigating new waters—all the while feeling less than well, either physically, emotionally, or both.

We are prime targets for those who are disreputable and looking to make a quick buck off desperate people. The primary thing to remember is that *there is no quick fix for Lyme disease.*

Using that as a measuring stick, the medical consumer must be on the alert for:

▪ *Any remedy billed as a "cure."* There is no such thing at this time. If there were, you can bet that major companies would be advertising, producing, and disseminating it worldwide with the blessings of reputable clinicians and researchers.

▪ *Remedies available only online, through mail order or one source, or those that contain "secret ingredients."* This should make you suspicious immediately. Furthermore, remember that there is only one "cure" for Lyme disease—killing the spirochete—and that requires antibiotics.

▪ *Doctors who advertise on billboards or in other splashy media.* Often, these doctors present case history testimonials but little in the way of research or substance. They rely on personality and advertising instead of solid therapeutic procedures and care.

▪ *Pseudo–Lyme disease hot lines.* Some hot lines truly provide solid information and referral services—if they're backed by a reputable nonprofit organization (e.g., the Lyme Disease Association or the Lyme Disease Network). Some, however, are funded by companies seeking to be paid for such referrals, and may, in fact, give you the name of only one doctor—possibly the one who started the hot line. Others are just come-ons for donations, which they request with every button option. You should not pay for simple information. Call your local Lyme support group or hospital as an alternative if a call to a "hot line" seems bogus.

▪ *Practitioners of any sort who encourage total dependence upon them for your wellness.* Whether from the medical mainstream or from alternative medical therapies, the reputable physician will assist you to independent wellness. Anyone encouraging dependence is more interested in your pocketbook than in your health.

Traditionally, medical doctors have concerned themselves only with the pathology of illness, treatment of the patient's symptoms, and resolution of the signs of disease. Today, many of those who are treating Lyme disease—itself out of the mainstream disease path—recognize that medical science does not have all the answers and that adjunctive therapies, including new ways of eating, exercising, and reducing stress, may be just as important to the patient's recovery as the antibiotics prescribed (see chapter 3).

Throw into the equation the success of medical treatments from other cultures, the need to treat the total person since Lyme disease is a multisystemic infection, and the desire and need for patients to take an active role in the process, and you have an approach to Lyme disease that is best termed "multimodal therapy."

LYME DISEASE REHABILITATION

Dr. Joseph Burrascano of Long Island has been treating Lyme disease patients since the mid-1980s, although he says he has suffered with it since his own teenage years. He is a physician who has crossed that researcher-clinician barrier—as involved in research as most academics, yet treating a battalion of Lyme patients from an assortment of states across the country. His treatment procedures are based upon years of studying, refining, and practicing what he preaches.

"Those with long-standing Lyme end up in poor physical condition. Even with successful treatment of the Lyme infection, they will not return to normal unless they take an active role in personal rehabilitation," says Burrascano.

In the later stages of Lyme, muscles may spasm and atrophy; the heart muscle suffers; the joints, nerves, and liver are negatively affected; and the patient's overall stamina and immune system suffer. As a result, Lyme patients become weak and tired and are at increased risk for heart attack and diabetes.

Burrascano maintains that physical therapy, particularly aerobics after the patient's stamina begins to increase, plays an important

role in the patient's recovering his or her health. Particularly
with late-stagers, this therapy should be very individualized.

"One hundred percent of those who went into an aggressive
rehabilitation program got better. It has a positive impact on
reversing the effects of Lyme disease. I usually recommend that a
patient begin slowly, and that immediately after exercising, they
take a very hot bath and then nap. As the weeks go by, they won't
need the nap and will gradually increase their level of activity."

Apart from the gradual strengthening of the overall body system, another reason that aerobics works for the Lyme patient is
that it increases the blood flow and body temperature—a setting
in which the spirochete cannot thrive.

HYPERBARIC OXYGEN THERAPY

Anyone who ever watched a Jacques Cousteau scuba-diving
special is probably familiar with hyperbaric chambers. The wiry
exploration diver would ominously warn that one of his divers
had gone down too deep, absorbed too much nitrogen, and had
gotten the "bends." A flurry of excitement would accompany
hauling the limp diver out of the water and placing him in what
looked like a room-sized steel vault while the pressure inside the
chamber was increased and then gradually decreased so as to
"bring the diver up" naturally, allowing sedentary gases like
nitrogen to bleed off, replaced by life-giving oxygen.

Since the 1980s, however, hyperbaric chambers, which
deliver pure oxygen under pressure to the red blood cells and
organs in the body, have been utilized by the medical profession
to assist in healing a wide variety of conditions, ranging from gas
gangrene to burns. This type of focused treatment was found to
accelerate recovery.

In 1998, Dr. William Fife, of Texas A&M's Hyperbaric Laboratory, broke new ground with his study demonstrating that HBO
therapy affected *Borrelia burgdorferi* spirochetes in patients with
Lyme disease. While pure oxygen inhaled at ground-level pressure does not affect the spirochetes, HBO therapy forces oxygen

into the body's blood and cells, creating a toxic environment in which the spirochete cannot live—but does not harm its human host. In fact, the exciting part of the experiment is that while most antibiotics cannot attack spirochetes in the brain because they cannot cross the blood-brain barrier, the pressurized oxygen can.

Today, hyperbaric chambers in New York, Florida, and Texas, among other places, have opened their doors to treating Lyme in addition to a host of other illnesses. It is important, however, to know what you are getting into—literally. Ask all the right questions, says Dr. Glenn Butler, of Mt. Vernon Hospital's Hyperbaric Medicine department. Butler knows whereof he speaks. Trained as a chemical engineer and cofounder of the Professional Diving School of New York, which has trained thousands of commercial divers for posts such as oil rigs in the North Sea, Butler's hospital office sports mechanical designs and drawings of his newest refinements to the standard hyperbaric chamber. His focus is now utilizing the familiar chamber to go where no medicine has gone before.

Like most things that have evolved over the last fifteen years, the modern HBO chamber is smaller and sleeker, looking more like a bullet-shaped glass space capsule in which a patient can recline, watch television, or listen to music during therapy. It is here that Lyme patients, among others, lie down for approximately ninety minutes every other day, for a prescribed number of weeks.

"You ask what does it feel like? You know how your ears pop when you go up in a plane?" says sixteen-year-old Conner, whose therapy so relieved his chronic Lyme symptoms that his parents purchased and refitted a used chamber in Florida, rather than continue to pay $250 per treatment. "It feels like the pressure is building and then you breathe in oxygen. The chamber helps my cognitive abilities. When I haven't done it in a while, I have more seizures, my memory goes. I get peripheral ghosts—a kind of translucent image in the right area of my eye."

The people who use the chamber and feel the effects love it. But there are many both in and out of the medical community who still view the benefits with a healthy skepticism. Currently, a study is being conducted by Butler in conjunction with Drs. Charles Pavia, Kenneth Liegner, and Zahid Niazi to study further the effectiveness of HBO therapy on the spirochete during infection. Butler cautions anyone thinking about investigating this type of symptom relief to do their homework before they open their wallets. "Just because a dive center may have a hyperbaric chamber, that doesn't mean they are qualified to give you medical assistance," he says. "This is an adjunctive medical treatment, first of all, to be used in conjunction with antibiotic therapy, not in place of it. Secondly, here are some of the things Butler says you should check out:

- Does the center have certified technicians?
- Does the center have a physician in attendance at all times, particularly during treatments?
- Will the physician conduct a complete physical examination for contraindications (such as a lung defect) and do a chest X ray and blood workup?
- What is the treatment protocol? Butler has found that two and a half atmospheres (or 82.5 feet of pressure) for ninety minutes with a couple of air breaks to be effective, while guarding against any possibility of seizures. Beware of the center that tells you that they take you down to two atmospheres for an hour. This is ineffective for anything other than relieving you of your money.
- What type of follow-up does the center provide? "If a patient doesn't get a Herxheimer-like reaction, I'd be very suspicious," says Butler. "Either the dosage is too low or Lyme disease is not involved. I can't stress strongly enough that this must be supervised by a Lyme-literate physician." Cost of one HBO session will run anywhere from $125 to $250 at an independent center and up to $500 per treatment at a hospital. And no, insurance will not cover the treatment.

CHIROPRACTIC AND KINESIOLOGY

Mention the word "stress" to most people and they will immediately think of a weekend with unfavorite relatives, a job deadline, or financial or relationship problems. This is emotional stress, but doctors look at three other types of stressors, including physical, biochemical, and thermal.

Lyme disease patients suffer all four kinds of stress, yet antibiotic therapy addresses only the biochemical, and in doing so, causes further chemical stress to the body. For that reason, many Lyme patients are finding that chiropractic, kinesiology, and acupuncture—all of which are designed to realign the body's various energy systems—have not only provided relief of symptoms, but also assisted in boosting the body's immune system.

Dr. Edward Burstein is one of only 117 diplomates of the International College of Applied Kinesiology worldwide. The founder of Berkeley Heights Chiropractic Center, in a Lyme-endemic area of New Jersey, he is a board-certified teacher and has lectured at numerous hospitals on immune, autoimmune, and chronic degenerative diseases. He is also seeing an increasing number of Lyme patients.

"Lyme disease seems to attack the weakest systems in a person's body. We see many, many people with Lyme, and every single person is different," says Burstein. "We need to tune up each person to as high a functioning level as possible.

"When the body is in a stressed state, many physiological changes take place. Blood pressure goes up, digestion slows, and muscles tense—all of the body's systems are on alert to deal with the stress. Continued distress is harmful because the body becomes exhausted from working overtime. If the stress is emotional or biochemical in nature, and continues, the resistance phase begins; the body attempts to adapt to the stress. This phase can go on for a long time and eventually the body weakens.

"The last phase is exhaustion or burnout," says Burstein. "The body no longer has the energy to contain the stress and begins to break down. Expressed as chronic fatigue, this phase is probably the most universal in our society."

This breakdown of the body's natural defenses complicates both the treatment for and the recovery from Lyme disease in that it can mask other problems. Harry, a fifty-year-old designer and avid jogger, was in a disseminated stage of Lyme before he was diagnosed. By that time, he could hardly get out of bed. Still symptomatic after fourteen months on antibiotics, he sought an adjunctive therapy. It was discovered that not only did he have a parasite in his intestine, but there was mercury in his system as well, which contributed to his swollen knees. Two months of treatment cleared up both problems, and his body began to reclaim its strength and his Lyme symptoms diminished.

The emphasis, once again, is on a multimodal approach to attacking Lyme. Straight medical treatment may not relieve all symptoms, and straight chiropractic may not either. If you are inclined to employ an adjunctive therapy, you should look for a medical doctor, osteopath, or chiropractor who practices applied kinesiology. This is a system that not only evaluates the body's structural, chemical, and mental aspects, but also utilizes nutrition, diet, acupressure (similar to acupuncture but without needles), and exercise to revive the total person.

A reputable practitioner will perform a number of noninvasive diagnostic medical tests before recommending a specific treatment path.

HOMEOPATHY

Another version of natural healing as an adjunctive therapy is homeopathy, which was begun in the early 1800s by German physician Samuel Hahnemann. His beliefs that "like cures like" and that medicines become more potent as they are diluted have given rise to a whole field of noninvasive therapy that has ardent detractors as well as ardent followers—including the British royal family, which has had a homeopathic doctor on staff since the time of Queen Victoria.

Much of homeopathy includes solid nutrition and lifestyle practices, and for those doctors like David Frerking, of Tavares, Florida, who are seeing an increasing number of Lyme patients, it is part of a multimodal attack on the disease.

"My approach is not to treat Lyme specifically, but to treat the entire body after performing a number of diagnostic tests," says Frerking, a member of the Board of Chiropractic Diagnosis and Preventive Medicine. "Traditional medicine says we must control the body; chiropractic philosophy says our bodies know how to be healthy and control themselves. When that's interfered with, the body's ability to function breaks down.

"Antibiotics given for Lyme disease push the organism into the cells. Homeopathics draws it out into the bloodstream where the body can find it. The substances used in homeopathy are diluted to stimulate the body to enhance its own response to fight off infection."

ELECTROMAGNETIC MACHINES

Dan Tracey of Speculator, New York, thought there had to be a better way to help his wife get through the Lyme hell of antibiotics, relapses, and twenty-one months of disorientation. In 1994, he delved into various scientific theories and gradually constructed a machine based on the works of inventor Rolle Reife. The result of his work is a unit that operates on the theory that every living cell has an electric frequency. By destroying the cell's electric frequency, you kill the offending cell. So far, many people swear by the results and EM machines are being utilized throughout the country to combat a variety of ills from cancer to arthritis to severe allergies.

"It's not a cure," he emphasizes, "but it helps." Treatments last from one to three minutes and must be repeated until complete relief is attained. Patients wishing to try this type of treatment may be able to get information on the location of the nearest generator from their Lyme support group.

The important things to remember when seeking adjunctive therapies for Lyme disease are caution and common sense. Many feel, however, that they don't know where to turn for adequate information and assume that, if something was important for the public to know, the health department would be the first to tell them. In most cases, they assume too much.

20.

Practical Prevention and Public Health

The U.S. Department of Defense takes Lyme and other tick-borne diseases so seriously that it now manufactures uniforms that are impregnated with repellent. The army equips field soldiers with an infrared device in each helmet whereby troops can be deployed to avoid high tick-infestation areas. Yet the state of California, which has had approximately 30,000 cases of Lyme disease in 2001–2002, doesn't have a single article warning the public about Lyme disease on its state health department website.

Public health officials from across the country complain that budget cutbacks leave little funding for the protection of the public, let alone dollars for education and prevention of Lyme, yet the federal government allocated $31 million for two years in a row to study West Nile virus, which had infected only 153 people by August of 2003.

Ovid, that ancient Roman who held some minor government positions before retiring to write poetry, might not have anticipated Lyme disease when he penned his often quoted and paraphrased line "The best defense is a good offense," but it has become the battle cry of those in the Lyme arena. The surest "cure" for Lyme disease is protection and education, and this must occur in three areas: your own person, home, and community.

Because Lyme disease is a very real environmental hazard and has a negative impact on the health of an area, people are beginning to become paranoid about participating in activities they formerly enjoyed. Many have given up camping, hiking, jogging, fishing, hunting, or even picnicking, especially in Lyme-endemic areas. Parents have forbidden their children to go out and play in the yard, go on school field trips to recreational areas, or leave the house unless covered from head to toe with clothing. And some health department officials attempt to walk a fine line between animal rights activists who protest deer hunting and frightened citizens who would like to wipe out any population of animals that might carry the infected ticks.

The problem with all of these anxious approaches is that they are treating the symptom and not the problem. Like the citizen who puts bars on his windows and does not go outside because of increase in crime in the neighborhood, some citizens are becoming prisoners in their own homes and offices because of the danger of Lyme disease.

The problem is the infected tick and the solution is eradication. *This* is where a major emphasis of education and protection must be—not on the elimination of activities. Once again, the solution is available, but it is up to each of us to implement it personally and demand its implementation on community and statewide levels.

PERSONAL PROTECTION

Most of us who have had any contact with Lyme disease, either personally or through the media, are familiar with the warning to wear long pants tucked into socks, long-sleeved shirts, gloves, and goggles, if possible. While this is ideal, and may discourage a tick from getting to one's skin, the image of having to bundle up during hot weather spells, when tick infestation is highest, may have a reverse effect on the public's motivation. Shorts, T-shirts, and bathing suits are here to stay, so other precautions against tick bites also need to be taken.

The following guidelines for personal protection against tick bites should be followed particularly in those areas in which Lyme is endemic and especially during the months of May through October.

- Don't walk barefoot or in open sandals outside. In Lyme-endemic areas, even short grass can harbor infected ticks.
- Since feet, ankles, and legs are primary points of contact, do wear long pants if walking through woods or tall grasses. Likewise, a hat is advisable if you are going to be in the woods or tall vegetation.
- Use a DEET-type repellent on exposed skin or on clothing or camping gear if outdoor activities are going to be prolonged. Since repellents on skin are potentially neurotoxic, spraying something like Permanone on the clothes and equipment may be better tolerated.
- Wear light-colored clothing so ticks will be more visible upon inspection.
- Check yourself every several hours during a long outing, and even more thoroughly upon returning home, preferably while you are still outside. Remember to look in those areas where ticks like to hide: the base of the neck, waistbands and/or brassieres, under arms, behind the knees, around ankles, in underwear and pubic hair.
- Take any clothing worn and throw it into the dryer for fifteen minutes on high heat. This will kill any ticks on the clothes. (Ticks have been known to live underwater for days, so putting the clothes in the washing machine will be ineffective.)
- Shower and brush hair thoroughly to discourage the attachment of any ticks.
- If you go outside to carry firewood into the house, consider using a repellent-sprayed carrier instead of holding the wood against your body.
- If camping, spray your equipment and tent with an effective repellent (see page 239) that lasts for up to forty-eight hours. When changing clothes, seal those that have been worn in a plastic bag until you can get them home to put in the dryer.
- Hunters and trappers should hang animal carcasses away from human activity for at least twelve hours so that ticks have a chance to drop off. In order to prevent the ticks from simply dropping off and crawling away, place a bucket of water with a concentration of liquid bleach directly under the carcass to kill falling

ticks. If the carcass is being dressed in the field, it is advisable to wear rubber gloves to minimize chances of infection.

- Inspect your children daily for ticks and/or teach them to inspect themselves, particularly in "private" areas of their bodies.
- If you do find a tick, do not panic. Also, do not use a cigarette, petroleum jelly, nail polish, kerosene, or a match to remove it. This will only cause the tick to inject more "poison" into your system. Grasp the tick with fine tweezers, as close to the skin as possible, and pull gently, straight out. You can then place the tick in a small plastic bag or other container with a blade of grass or some moist cotton and take it to your doctor or health department for testing. If you live in a Lyme-endemic area, contact your internist and report the tick bite to him. If he or she cannot be reached, consider going to the hospital emergency room.
- Check your pets for ticks (see chapter 13).
- Keep pets that have had possible tick exposure outdoors off the furniture, particularly any bedding.

USING REPELLENTS

Few people would advocate spraying chemicals needlessly on the human body, but it is generally accepted that the dangers of Lyme disease warrant the added protection of safe tick repellents. The most effective repellent that can be safely applied to the skin contains a component known as DEET.

Developed originally for use in the military during the 1950s, DEET is now applied more than an estimated 400 million times a year. A five-year compilation of data from the American Association of Poison Control Centers showed products containing DEET to be relatively safe, and it is approved for use by the Environmental Protection Agency (EPA). In carefully controlled independent tests using mosquitoes and human subjects, as reported in the July 4, 2002, edition of the *New England Journal of Medicine,* insect repellents containing DEET provided better protection from bites for longer periods than other widely used repellent products. DEET disrupts the ability of biting insects to detect the source of carbon dioxide—the gas naturally given off by our skin and in our breath—which is what attracts mosquitoes, ticks, and other insects to us. Insects aren't killed—they just can't locate their prey for a period of hours.

Parents should apply DEET-based repellents to younger children (rather than allow them to do it themselves) by placing a small amount of the repellent on your hands and then rubbing the repellent on the child's face and exposed neck. Be careful not to apply repellent to the hands or any other part of the body that may wind up in the little one's mouth.

Several of the more popular and effective products manufactured with DEET include the Repel line from Wisconsin Pharmacal Company, which produces several products in varying strengths for specific purposes, Deep Woods Off, and Ultrathon from 3M, which in tests conducted by *Consumer Reports* repelled ticks for up to ten hours.

It is important to remember that the manufacturer's instructions should be carefully read and followed prior to use. There is no need to "take a bath" in the repellent, and it should be applied in a well-ventilated area. Inhaling fumes or overspraying can result in adverse reactions, and repellent should never be sprayed over cut or broken skin.

A repellent that was tested by the military, particularly in Saudi Arabia, and found to be 100 percent effective in killing and repelling ticks is Permethrin. It is commercially available in an aerosol spray under the names Repel, Permanone, Permethrin, and Duranon. A single application to clothing or equipment is effective for up to two days. Remember that safe application consists of spraying the clothing while it is *off* the body, then allowing it to dry in a well-ventilated area before wearing.

MAKE YOUR HOME UNINVITING

Making one's home a castle usually involves investing hours and dollars in landscaping, ornamental walks and walls, and lawn maintenance. Unfortunately, not only do humans find shrubs, hanging vines, and trees inviting, so do ticks.

In a CDC study of four hundred properties in upstate New York, several common factors were revealed. According to Dr. Durland Fish, associate professor and director of the Lyme Disease Center for New York Medical College:

- Tick infestation was seven times higher in those areas that were unmaintained (i.e., woods, borders, or "natural" landscaping).

- Stone walls are favorite places for ticks to congregate, so humans should avoid sitting on or working around them during those times of year when nymphal ticks are active.

- Ticks love ornamental shrubs.

- Insecticide application of Sevin (carbaryl), Dursban (chlorpyrifos), and Permethrin was 97 percent effective in controlling ticks for the entire nymphal season. Although the Permethrin worked the best, it is not available in all states. Both Sevin and Dursban are commonly used, both on lawns and in a number of pet products, with good safety records. The granular form of the insecticides was more effective on lawns, which are not critical habitats for wildlife.

Sensitive to public criticism of the use of pesticides, Fish says, "You have a choice between being exposed to insecticides or Lyme disease. It's your decision.

"Remember, it's not the ticks that you find that are the ones likely to give you trouble. They are the failures, the losers. The successful ticks are the ones you don't see."

There are several other home-based strategies that can be employed to reduce the risk of tick attraction. One method is to increase the lawn size, pushing trees, ornamentals, and hedges away from the house. Since open lawn has the lowest rate of tick infestation across the board, cutting back on the number of shade trees, particularly those close to the house, will reduce your risk.

Dr. Kirby Stafford, chief scientist in Connecticut's department of forestry and horticulture, also suggests laying a three-foot wide wood-chip border separating woods, stone walls, shrubby areas, and tall grass. His research showed that this border resulted in about 50 percent fewer ticks on the lawn. Other tips include cleaning out leaf litter at the edge of the property and stone walls, a move that results in a 70 percent reduction in the tick population on your lawn.

Bird-watching is fun, but with ten billion migrating birds carrying untold billions of ticks, is it really that important to you? Get rid of those birdhouses and bird-feeders from your trees and then tune in to Animal Planet on cable for a bird fix.

It is wise to locate children's sandboxes and swing sets in open, sunny areas rather than shady ones. A large beach umbrella raised during sandbox play will protect little ones from the sun's harmful rays, yet allow you to keep the unit in an area unattractive to ticks.

Finally, go after the mouse population, which serves as an important host for ticks. Not only are the mice carriers during the summer months, but when the weather turns cold they tend to run for nice warm houses—bringing their ticks with them.

TARGETING TICKS

Aiming to control the ticks that feed on mice, Harvard University researchers developed Damminix. This is cotton soaked with Permethrin and packed in biodegradable tubes that are placed around a specific property. The mice collect the cotton, take it back to their nests for building material, and kill ticks in the process. This has been shown to be effective, but it must be widely used in a given geographic location to have a major impact.

Two other strategies are proving highly effective in reducing the tick populations:

■ The Four-Poster—Developed by scientists at the Agricultural Research Station in Kerrville, Texas, this consists of a bin filled with corn and vertical paint rollers that have been laced with a tick-killing agent. When the deer come to the bin to feed, they must brush their heads against the rollers, which passively apply the "tickacide." Tested at sites from Massachusetts to Maryland for four years by the U.S. Food and Drug Administration, the Four-Poster has been shown to reduce the ticks carried by deer anywhere from 69 to 80 percent.

▪ The Tick-Force Management System—Otherwise known as the Bait Box, this was developed by the CDC, which holds the patent along with Aventis, to control the ticks on small rodents. As with the Four-Poster, the rodent comes to the box to feed and its coat is brushed with a dose of Fipronil, the same chemical which in trials has been shown to control ticks on dogs and cats for up to forty-two days. Both the Four-Poster and the Bait Box will be available through the American Lyme Disease Foundation (see appendix C).

Other research moving forward includes an exploration of two types of fungi that kill ticks (conducted at the University of Florida) and a study of the use of pheromones to attract ticks toward a pesticide that would kill them.

Personal protection, becoming conscientious about your property, and targeting ticks through new scientific devices are an excellent start to preventing Lyme disease. These methods, however, will not do the job unless we bring both the problem and the solution to the attention of those in our cities and states who have the power to implement important community protection programs.

COMMUNITY PROTECTION: A TAXPAYER'S RIGHT

Many citizens only come in contact with their state's health department via unsafe restaurants, school health rules, or travel plans that require immunizations. Good medical consumers, however, should know what their health department is doing in the areas of environmental hazards, disease control, and education. After all, they are paying for these services through tax dollars.

Two outstanding groups, the Rhode Island State Department of Health and STOP—Stop Ticks On People—in Dutchess County, New York, have been leading the way in focusing public and governmental attention on Lyme disease. They take a two-prong approach to attack the problem at the source: enacting measures to get rid of disease-bearing ticks and educating the public. They have raised the bar on what public health entities can do with input from concerned private citizens and cooperation from elected officials.

Jill Auerbach had been a programmer with IBM for years when she began her own descent into Lyme. Her body and mind failing her, but too embarrassed to say anything at work, her Lyme went undiagnosed, then was misdiagnosed as lupus, before she finally saw a Lyme-literate physician. An activist by nature, Auerbach spent the next six years bringing Lyme to the attention of city and county committee members. Not difficult to do, she says, since Dutchess County has the highest level of infected ticks in the country per capita. What the Dutchess County Department of Health and the Hudson Valley Lyme Disease Committee began to focus on was the source of the problem—the ticks.

"We finally realized the answer is not in treating us or vaccinating us; it's getting rid of all the ticks," says Auerbach. "We had been tackling this from the wrong end. We started focusing on the environment. No matter what else, there shouldn't be any fractionalization when it comes to the environment." The result was the formation of STOP through an affiliation with United Way of Dutchess County, the Lyme Disease Association, the American Lyme Foundation, and the Dutchess County Task Force to Reduce Ticks and Lyme Disease. STOP formed both a scientific advisory board as well as a community advisory board and has obtained funding from the CDC to continue researching environmental methods of reducing the tick population while educating the public. When it comes to stopping Lyme, Auerbach doesn't take no for an answer. When she expressed concern over area children playing in an unsprayed and unprotected school yard and was told by school officials there was no problem, she took a piece of dry ice on a board and placed it on the playground. Within hours, the ice and board were covered with ticks—and school officials paid attention.

STOP has produced educational materials and an informative website and made public health its mission. "There are methodologies to reducing the tick population, but there is generally no funding for it," Auerbach says. "It is up to us to start making noise to our federal legislators that we want an effective means to reduce ticks."

In Rhode Island, the Governor's Commission on Lyme and Other Tick-Borne Diseases was responsible for passing groundbreaking legislation (see chapter 17) regarding the diagnosis, treatment, and insurance coverage of Lyme disease. But activities concerning public education have fallen to the Department of Health, headed by Dr. Patricia Nolan, assisted by Helen Drew. Nolan noted that a major issue in Rhode Island's new unwanted status of having the second highest infection rate of Lyme and other tick-borne diseases in the country "was the public's lack of awareness of the severity of Lyme. Individuals need to be aware of just how damaging Lyme can be to their health so that they will take more active precautions to avoid tick bites," she says. And the only way for a state health department to move a program like this forward is to make it a priority by understanding the millions of dollars lost each year when citizens become ill with Lyme.

Recommendations for public health that are currently being implemented include the dissemination of information to both children and parents regarding personal protection at schools, camps, day care, parks, and other child-centered programs. State employees who work outdoors are considered "high risk" and an information program specifically for them is being designed. Towns are also being encouraged to develop strategies to limit tick contact with humans.

Some people feel that looking out for the public's health isn't just the province of state health departments but should be reflected by other health professionals as well. Frank Corvino, president and CEO of Greenwich Hospital, says that a hospital is part of the community it serves and, as such, has a responsibility to address community needs. The one-hundred-year-old hospital, which is undergoing a $99 million face-lift and expansion, has put its "we want to be a healing center" philosophy into action. From the classical music and waterfall in the high-ceilinged lobby—"Going to the hospital is never pleasant," says Corvino, "so we try to provide a warm and calming atmosphere"—to a full schedule of community meetings, task forces, and support groups, area residents need only ask for the hospital's help to get a quick response.

"We see Lyme disease as a real threat to the well-being of area residents and our hospital as a major player in keeping them well, not just taking care of those who get sick," says Corvino. "For that reason, we have co-sponsored educational seminars, supported fund-raising events in a meaningful way as a patron, and lent our name and credibility to a task force."

Integral to a Lyme disease education project is a cooperative relationship with the local media. Approach the editors of local newspapers, develop a relationship with science or community reporters, and don't forget any local radio or television stations. This is a partnership that can help each party.

Not all health departments are sympathetic to the Lyme disease situation for various reasons, but that should not stop the public from taking action. If you are turned away by your health department, seek out a sympathetic and knowledgeable internist or other medical professional to assist in setting up a program. Every state has some facility already in place that people can utilize as a satellite. Sometimes it's a medical school or a medical center. Find out who is in charge of infectious diseases and talk to that person.

The politics of public health would tend to downplay anything that would upset the status quo. Public health service is traditionally a conservative wing which is why it is important to have those numbers—of ticks, infected people, actual cases. It sets up some credibility. The public health departments set the tone for local physicians, and they have a responsibility to educate those physicians. If the physician gets a signal to either worry or not worry about a particular matter, that impression can last a long time. In the meantime, new facts may come to light that need to be passed on. This is an ongoing process. And a very important one.

WHAT HAPPENED TO THE VACCINE?

For a generation that is accustomed to simply getting a vaccination to keep serious diseases at bay, there is a learning curve at work in dealing with Lyme disease. Not since the spirochetal research involving syphilis has medical science come up against an organism as frighteningly brilliant and devious as the spirochete that carries Lyme. The comfortable, familiar approach to dealing with disease has to be set aside.

A vaccine, by definition, is a preparation of a weakened or killed pathogen, such as a bacterium or virus, or a portion of the pathogen's structure that, upon injecting it into the human body, creates an antibody response but does not cause infection or disease. The problem with Lyme disease, as we have discovered over the years, is that the spirochete not only does not behave like other pathogens, it continually mutates. And once it is in the human body, it has a party replicating, hiding—and infecting. Since most vaccines are developed in laboratories under strict and limited guidelines, attempts at creating a successful vaccine against Lyme disease—all strains of Lyme disease—has so far been a disappointment.

The first Lyme vaccine, Lymerix, manufactured by Glaxo-SmithKline, was pulled off the market at the FDA's direction in 2002 due to increasing reports that the vaccine itself was causing Lyme-like arthritic and neurologic symptoms in those who had received it. The government's database of possible side effects of Lymerix lists 640 emergency room visits, 34 life-threatening reactions, 77 hospitalizations, 198 disabilities, and

6 deaths after people took the shots since the CDC endorsed it. Hundreds of class action lawsuits sealed the vaccine's fate.

Another vaccine has been in development for the last ten years. Researchers at SUNY Stony Brook and Brookhaven National Laboratory have been looking at the crystal structure of the proteins on the surface of *Borrelia* attempting to develop a product that would be effective against all strains of Lyme. This vaccine, according to a spokesperson at Baxter International, which has licensed the patent, may still be years away from hitting the market.

The best protection against Lyme disease and other tick-borne illnesses remains first, prevention, and second, a rapid diagnosis and aggressive treatment.

As has been said by those toiling in the Lyme field, the ultimate responsibility for education and activism is in the hands of those affected by the disease. Enlightened health officials and doctors can do only so much: the driving force for change must be the public. This realization has fueled the formation of growing numbers of support groups, coalitions, and political entities.

21.

Support and Activism: A Vital Link

To see what is right and not to do it is want of courage.

—Confucius, *Analects*

Prior to the Civil War, one of the most organized support networks was established in the United States. It was called the Underground Railroad. Although it was neither a railroad nor underground, it provided runaway slaves with information, contacts, and a helping hand to freedom. And it provided more; it let them know that they were not alone in their plight and that there were many who would risk their own safety and livelihood to do the right thing.

Today, another type of "underground railroad" is in effect across the country, and its mission is not terribly unlike its predecessor's. Along this network, Lyme disease patients can find information, names of doctors who are brave enough to treat them, sympathy, and encouragement in their flight to freedom from a disease that can enslave both the mind and the body. And they, too, are finding more than they expected.

In order to be heard above the din of needy voices and the kaleidoscope of demands pelting our nation's medical establishment and its lawmakers, these Lyme disease patients, doctors, and advocates are developing networks of political activism. From California to Wisconsin to New England to Florida, support groups have been activated, coalitions formed, independent projects undertaken, and legislation written, all in the name of freedom from Lyme. And as surely as the Underground Railroad crystallized the polarity of the country regarding slavery, the exploding Lyme disease movement promises to forge a new look at health care and patients' rights in the face of massive bureaucratic denial and lethargy.

FINDING SUPPORT, FINDING SANITY

They walk in gingerly the first time, some shuffling slowly, some leaning on canes, family members, or walkers. Most are desperate—ill, depressed, financially strained, and frustrated over a medical enigma that has infected the whole family's psyche. And what they find at the Lyme support group meeting is more than they had hoped for: reassurance that they are not alone or crazy (despite the fact that several doctors might have told them they were); education about this complex disease and avenues for treatment; and contact with others of every race, creed, and color who can offer practical methods of dealing with annoying symptoms that well-meaning but inexperienced doctors cannot provide.

Whether you're speaking with Marvina Lodge or Richard Goldman in Florida, Phyllis Mervine in California, or Diane Blanchard and Debbie Siciliano in Connecticut, you hear that their reasons for starting a support group were the same: anger and frustration. Anger at members of the medical profession for abdicating their responsibility to teach the public about this disease and then reacting with arrogance when confronted by continual illness; and frustration over the isolation the illness imposes, the loss of control over one's body systems, and the emotional havoc it wreaks.

This was the situation in which Betty Gross found herself fifteen years ago, before many people had even heard of Lyme disease. Mother of four (two of whom are doctors) and a grandmother, she was a veteran of years of volunteer work with Girl Scouts, Twins Clubs, and special interest groups in her Westchester,

New York, community when she was hit with Lyme disease. Suddenly, folding a basket of laundry not only had to be planned, it exhausted her so badly that she needed a three-hour nap to recover. Searching for information regarding this strange illness that was sweeping through her community in 1988, she found little available. What she found were afflicted neighbors who would call and say, "Am I going to live through this?"

She turned to the county health department and volunteered her services to get information out to the community and the doctors. She involved the newspapers and local service groups. Each outreach brought a flood of response and need. After attending a leadership training course for support groups, she placed a small blurb in the local newspaper about the formation of a group for those involved in Lyme disease.

"We had to change our location twice even before that first meeting because the telephone calls in response to the newspaper ad were overwhelming," said Betty. "Finally, Reverend Charles Colwell of the Saint Barnabas Episcopal Church just told me to take over the whole church and it's a good thing he did."

More than seventy people packed the charming white colonial church that evening in 1988, and the first Lyme support group in the nation was established. Today, there are approximately 196 Lyme support groups in the United States and Canada. More are being formed quickly as people in states ranging from Maine to New Mexico and Kentucky to Arkansas find that they, too, are facing obstacles in obtaining a diagnosis and treatment for Lyme disease, Master's disease, Lyme-like illnesses, and a plethora of co-infections.

"No one can amply gauge when you 'hit bottom' in Lyme disease because it's different for each person," said Betty, who passed away much too soon in 2003, though her work and indomitable spirit live on. "No one has an idea of how Lyme is going to twist and mangle your existence until it happens. People have to plumb the depths of themselves to deal with this. When a person contracts Lyme, their whole family becomes infected. When it is a child, other children in the family become invisible

under the impact of this disease. And Lyme makes people paranoid because of the reactions of those around them. We've had
a number of professionals who didn't want their colleagues to
know they had Lyme disease because the public hears syphilis
and Lyme mentioned in the same sentence and they mentally
connect the two diseases and avoid the Lyme patient."

Confidentiality is what a support group has going for it. As a
leader, you become privy to people's confidences, a private sur-
rendering of one's self as they share their feelings, their agonies,
and their worries. If anyone thinks they would like to start a
group, be prepared to keep these confidences locked up inside—
or don't do it.

Here is some further advice for those wishing to start a support group:

▪ Support groups need to be conduits of information. Evaluate the
doctors in the area and attempt to involve the enlightened ones. Then,
when the confidence of the group leaders is stronger, invite the other
doctors in the area.

▪ Being with your local health department, but don't rely solely on it.
Develop a relationship with the local media and exchange information.

▪ Bring in speakers from pharmaceutical companies dealing with
Lyme, legislators, and physicians, but leave time at meetings for people
to network and share their feelings and experiences. This is an important aspect of the support group because it lets people know that they
are not as isolated as they think, either in their struggles or their emotional strain—and that there is hope.

▪ Contact your local hospital or medical center to see if they will
allow you to hold your meetings there. Be prepared to teach the educational director about Lyme disease and how big a problem it presents
in your community. Go armed with facts, figures, and information as
well as a game plan for holding your meetings.

▪ If the hospital is unreceptive for any reason, contact your county
library for access to a meeting room. The library should have books on

Lyme disease on its shelves. If it doesn't, bring this matter to their attention. (You can begin with this latest edition of *Coping With Lyme Disease* by Denise Lang. Beware a brief volume under this title that was used, unauthorized, by a Maryland writer; there is no connection between the two books!)

▪ Prior to your first meeting, contact your local newspaper and speak to a reporter whose name you have seen on other health stories. Let him or her know about your meeting and that human interest stories are available. Newspapers are always looking for good health features that focus on readers in their circulation area. After your meeting, keep your health reporter informed of your progress and future speakers.

▪ Plan, if possible, to use a separate telephone line for handling calls about Lyme disease. Support group leaders have quickly found that their house and business lines can be tied up 24-7 with people needing help. Put basic information about your meetings, directions, and resource information on an outgoing message to prevent having to repeat yourself one hundred times.

"There is so much denial going on regarding Lyme disease, not just with doctors and government officials, but with the victims themselves," says Kathy Cavert, a registered nurse who founded the Midwest Lyme Disease Association. "People will justify all their symptoms by saying, 'Oh, I slept wrong, I'm under stress, I'm at that age when my body should be falling apart anyway' (this from people in their thirties and forties!). People have to be educated so they can get well.

"This disease isn't hitting the couch potatoes of the country who sit in front of the television drinking beer," says Cavert. "It's hitting the most active, brightest *doers*, and it is forcing them to have to reframe their whole existence in order to survive."

"A large part of what we do is information and support, and this becomes a full-time job," says Marvina Lodge, who runs a support group just north of Orlando, Florida. "I would tell anyone wanting to start a group to make sure you have help, backup of some kind, and if you get informed doctors involved that's even better. Part of our problem here in Florida is that we have hundreds upon hundreds of people infected and the doctors don't know anything about it; patients have to go out of state for treatment."

Lora Mermin, in Madison, Wisconsin, experienced the same type of situation when she was first infected in 1987. By 1988, a small ad placed in the local newspaper brought a half-dozen people to an informational meeting of what is now the Lyme Resource Group of Madison and South Central Wisconsin. Inspired by the hunger for information, Lora formed the Lyme Disease Education Project and combined informative issues of Lyme support group newsletters from across the country and published them under one cover. She, too, recognizes the need for people to reach out and make contact with those who can understand the Lyme experience. "We have some people who drive for two hours to get to our meetings. People are eager to talk; they need to know that they aren't crazy and that there is help available to them."

A number of the older and more active support groups have been the birthplaces of monthly newsletters that provide information and hope to thousands across the country (see appendix D), and a few more have made the transitions into the national arena.

The Lyme Disease Network, established by Carol and Bill Stolow in reaction to their young daughters' infection with Lyme, was one of the first to establish an information line for physicians across the country who want to know more about Lyme disease. Today, the Lyme Disease Network, which is affiliated with the Lyme Disease Association (LDA), not only offers an opportunity for physicians and Lyme victims to get the latest information but has spearheaded such creative efforts as getting local milk companies to put Lyme information on their milk cartons at critical times of the year.

THE INDEPENDENT ACTIVISTS

Fred Lawson was just a fifteen-year-old Louisiana boy when he suffered such severe head trauma in an accident that he officially died. His experience as he traveled back to life, to the hospital room where his body lay, led him to the knowledge that he was put back on earth for a specific reason. After years of struggling to relearn the simplest speech and life skills, he was infected with Lyme disease.

Now in his fifties, Lawson, who resides in Leesburg, Florida, dedicates his life to providing support for those suffering with Lyme. This dedication has led him to organize a network of 250 volunteers to meet airplanes carrying Lyme patients from Florida to treatment in New York and New Jersey. It has led him to develop Lyme educational programs with former Rams player Jim Youngblood and to speak nationally on the subject. He has also talked suicidal Lyme patients off roofs and found doctors for those in remote areas.

"It's so important that people work together—not against each other—to beat this disease," he says. "I've seen the devastation Lyme disease can cause; I've seen the pain and suffering, and I've been through it myself and am still going through it. Just about the time you think you have a handle on it, it comes at you from a different direction. People in this country are extremely ill and they need help. I know that this is why I was put back on earth, and I'll do what little I can to educate people about Lyme."

Several movie producers who were touched by Lyme have also moved into the educational arena by developing independent projects designed to educate both citizens and lawmakers.

Steven Zimmer's successful documentary on AIDS, which was made into a major motion picture, paved the way for his project: *Lyme Disease—Time For Truth,* a moving look at those who suffer with the disease and those who are fighting for them. It is available on videocassette.

When Neil Goldstein moved from Southern California to Pennsylvania, he found himself infected with Lyme disease and with nowhere to turn for information. He, along with Amy Jones, formed the Lyme Project of Hudson Valley. Initially set up to launch a multimodal attack on the problem, the project initiated epidemiological studies, produced public television programs, and established a support group.

Vincent Sorrentino's involvement with Lyme disease occurred when he was approached about filming a video to be shown to lawmakers in the New Jersey legislature who were trying to determine whether insurance companies should be mandated to continue coverage of their patients with Lyme. Although he had produced numerous documentaries on various human conditions, Lyme affected him so deeply that he formed Lyme Awareness Productions with several Lyme support groups for continued work in this area. Involved in producing the television docudrama about Lyme entitled *The Hidden Epidemic,* Sorrentino interviewed a number of children with the disease and walked away shaken. "On top of the incredible pain they endure, these kids have lost their friends, fallen behind in school, and seen their dreams disappear. It's very important that we do everything possible to bring awareness to the effects that Lyme disease is having on kids."

Another creative contribution came from cable television show producer Mary Ann Shanahan who had previously directed the award-winning PBS documentary *Children and Asthma: A Matter of Life and Breath,* and hosts a weekly Connecticut show called *The Best of Health.* It was while she was researching a segment on Lyme disease that she "became fascinated with this tick-borne illness." The result was a sixty-minute documentary, in 2003, *Lyme Disease: A Guide to Prevention,* narrated by Oscar-winning actress Meryl Streep and funded through a grant from the Division of Vector-Borne Infectious Diseases. It, too, has deservedly won numerous awards.

ACTIVIST GROUPS

When New York congressman George Hochbrueckner began talking about Lyme disease, many of his colleagues thought he was talking about something that afflicted citrus fruit. As one of the primary forces behind passage of a bill that would allocate nearly a million dollars for the protection from and treatment of Lyme disease in our armed forces overseas, and of another bill, cosponsored by Congressman Joseph Lieberman of Connecticut, proposing a national Lyme Awareness Week, he has served as the inspiration for many who want to move the Lyme battle into the political spotlight.

New Jersey governor Christie Whitman was diagnosed with Lyme disease in 1996. She was treated promptly and recovered fully. It was an irony that in early 1992, then governor Jim Florio of New Jersey had approved the Governor's Lyme Advisory Council, the first such group in the nation, comprising a cross section of experts to make recommendations for combating the disease. Following closely was the formation of the New York Lyme Disease Coalition (New Jersey already had one), and similar moves in several other states, including Wisconsin, which began organizing their own coalitions to serve as umbrella organizations linking the diverse support groups for political clout.

Ken Fordyce, chairman of the New Jersey Governor's Advisory Council and longtime member of the New Jersey Lyme Disease Coalition, feels that organized, unified efforts are the only way anything will be accomplished in solving the Lyme puzzle. His group has immersed itself in everything from legislation to education to producing a position paper outlining the rights of patients and listing recommendations for action, which highlight the need for long-term treatment and drug studies.

"People need to become involved because nothing will be done unless they are," says Fordyce. "If AIDS hadn't come along, Lyme disease would be the hottest disease under discussion right now because, among other things, it's so chemically interesting. But getting to the heart of the problem goes back to territorial imperative—people stake out a position and then defend it to the death. Our job as medical consumers is to bombard them with the latest information available and push for action. We're talking about our lives here, and the lives of our children."

Children were the motivating force for Diane Blanchard and Debbie Siciliano of Greenwich, Connecticut, in 1998, when the two mothers—frightened by the deterioration of their children who had contracted Lyme, and frustrated by the obstacles to good diagnosis, treatment, and education—formed the Greenwich Lyme

Disease Task Force. They worked with other mothers, many of whom, like themselves, came from high-powered professional backgrounds but found that their credentials didn't matter when pitted against an invading spirochete. Blanchard and Siciliano's task force grew to include both a community and medical board of volunteer directors and changed its name to Time For Lyme, Inc. It has dedicated itself to a type of guerilla activism of the highest quality that has resulted in raising more than $1.5 million to help establish the Columbia University Lyme Disease Research Center; working with the state attorney general's office to restore mandatory laboratory reporting of Lyme disease (which was discontinued in 2003 due to the overwhelming numbers of residents reportedly infected); working with U.S. Senator Christopher Dodd to further develop Lyme disease education and prevention initiatives; creating a compact tick removal kit that has been distributed through the Red Cross to all schools requesting it for use both in school and on field trips; sponsoring numerous conferences and seminars for educators and health professionals; and producing an educational video, *Time For Lyme—The Students, the Educators, and Lyme Disease,* which was made available for distribution to school systems all over the country, in addition to a variety of educational publications.

"Fighting Lyme disease is a daily battle," says Blanchard. "The willful ignorance of many doctors is astounding. But through all this pain, I found a lifelong passion and a group of friends that will carry me every day of my life. When you fight together like this, you connect at such a gut level because you are worried about each other and each other's children. That is a huge motivation. We're worried about all the children."

Siciliano agrees, encouraging everyone who can, to become an activist. "Nobody is going to do this for us. We have been fortunate to affiliate with the Lyme Disease Association; that's opened some doors. But when you look at the effect of Lyme disease on our children—dropping twenty-five IQ points in many cases with neurological impairment—it is horrifying to think what it means to the future of our country. We have to make the legislators listen, and we have to educate the academics and the physicians."

Education on all fronts has been the hallmark of the Lyme Disease Association (LDA) since Pat Smith took the reins approximately ten years ago. From traveling all over the country to meet with physicians, researchers, and those wishing to start Lyme support groups to presenting educational seminars for congressmen, senators, and federal officials, to coordinating worldwide research and funneling it to our scientists and providing a network of assistance to the disparate Lyme organizations on this continent, Smith has been so all-present in every facet of Lyme activism both in this country and abroad that most people wonder when and if she sleeps. Under her leadership, the LDA has been instrumental in funding more than $1 million in much needed studies, research, and international and domestic conferences on Lyme for physicians, researchers, patients, and activists in the United States and Europe, as well as establishing the Columbia University Lyme Disease Research Center. They have also produced instructional videos and DVDs, as well as a variety of publications with target audiences as varied as children, educators and health professionals, and politicians.

"We've come a long way, but there's still so much to do at every turn," says Smith, who is also a founding member of the recently established International Lyme and Associated Diseases Society (ILADS). "I hear from at least one attorney a week who is dealing with insurance companies on behalf of sick patients who can't get their entitled coverage. Education is always the key. There are so many people so sick out there who don't know where to turn. We need to educate the health departments, the doctors. Then, if one of them refuses to acknowledge or treat Lyme, you have evidence that he or she is just ignoring it. They can't say they are ignorant anymore, so that creates a different level of liability.

"I think through the LDA's work, people are beginning to feel like they're a part of a larger mission," says Smith. "And doctors feel more comfortable tapping in to our information, resources, and network. This is the way it has to operate in order to get to the bottom of this disease."

A number of support groups, foundations, alliances, and coalitions have formed to jump into the battle against Lyme disease. As recognition of the disease spreads, many more will be formed. One word of caution to the newly involved is necessary.

Any cause attracts the entire spectrum of human personality, from the reticent to the fanatic, from the educated to the ignorant, from the altruistic to the greedy. Lyme disease is no exception. The vast majority of organizations and foundations are reputable, but the wise medical consumer will ask some tough questions based on common sense before donating money or following a leader into battle.

Those organizations that ask for your donation, even on a well-publicized national level, should be able to provide you with an annual report of how the money is spent as well as references that should be checked out. You do not have to pay for referrals to doctors or groups; these are free through the LDA or your support groups (see appendix B).

Finally, educate yourself as to the nature of the disease and the political structure of the battle, rather than blindly joining under any banner proclaiming "Lyme." Remember, you can make a difference. You are the *only* one who can make a difference, but only if you join the fight as an informed medical consumer, not merely a passionate one.

22.

Conclusion: A Challenge to Fight

During the 1962 Cuban missile crisis between the United States and the Soviet Union, President John F. Kennedy received two conflicting communications from Soviet premier Nikita Khrushchev. One contained terms that were acceptable, the other did not. Attorney General Robert Kennedy was credited with a diplomatic maneuver—later dubbed the "Trollope ploy," after a recurrent theme in Anthony Trollope's novels in which the girl interprets a squeeze of her hand as a proposal of marriage. Robert Kennedy's suggestion was to deal with the acceptable message only and to ignore the other. President Kennedy went on to accept Khrushchev's offer and then set forth his own ideas of what that offer really was.

There are many medical consumers who will maintain that their physicians, insurance companies, and health agencies are masters of Trollope's ploy when dealing with Lyme disease. These entities will accept those symptoms and statements that fit neatly into preconceived patterns and ignore others, substituting their own experience and ideas for the facts.

While this gambit may work in international negotiations, it subverts the doctor-patient relationship, delays or circumvents successful treatment, and contributes to the continued ill health of formerly talented and productive citizens.

I am a big fan of the funny papers and one of my favorites is *Hagar the Horrible* for its right-on-the-button philosophy of everyday life. One wonderful strip could have been inspired by a Lyme patient. The town's doctor has chased down the rotund

Viking Hagar and his wife, Helga, and admonishes them: "You should trust doctors more. . . . Our first rule is: 'Do No Harm.'" Whereupon Helga turns to Hagar and comments, "It worries me that they'd need a *rule* to figure that out!"

Two basic medical tenets are (1) patients want to get well, and (2) doctors want to heal. In dealing with Lyme disease, these two groups more than ever before are going to have to put aside traditional methodologies and attack the problem rather than each other. This can be accomplished through the following methods:

1. Citizens today must view themselves as medical consumers and take responsibility for both maintaining good health and for participating in their own medical treatment when ill. There is no excuse, with the amount of information available on the Internet, for being a helpless isolationist any longer. We are responsible for our own good health and that of our families.

2. Physicians need to keep an open mind—and open ears—when dealing with Lyme and other difficult diseases that may require more reliance on their own powers of deductive reasoning than on unreliable tests. Medicine is an art and a science. None of us can ignore the "art" aspect as we attempt to utilize the scientific principles.

3. As we are faced with a new era of "brilliant bugs," drug-resistant bacteria, and emerging virulent organisms, doctors from both Lyme disease polarities need to put petty rivalries aside and work together to attack this illness. This natural competition is being utilized by both government and private institutions to ignore the growing problem of Lyme disease. The bottom line is: The patient loses. And with the rapid spread of this illness, the very doctors who downplay the disease's prevalence could find themselves on the patient's end of the tongue depressor.

4. Ideally, the American Medical Association would work with the American Bar Association to draw up guidelines governing disease protocols and presenting a united front to the gigantic, multitrillion-dollar insurance industry. We are losing too many good and dedicated physi-

cians to greedy corporate bottom lines. There are also too many physicians on generous insurance company payrolls who let the truth—and patient wellness—get overshadowed by the color of money. Here is where the AMA could take a leadership role in limiting the involvement of its members for the good of the Hippocratic Oath—and the patients they are sworn to help.

5. Physicians must also become activists in order to help protect themselves, not just with outlandishly skyrocketing malpractice insurance rates (there's that entity again!) but also to protect their rights to practice medicine as they see fit, within the context of moral standards. Busy-ness is no longer an excuse; everyone is busy trying to make a living, raise a family, and stay healthy. We have to work in a united partnership to protect each other.

It is only through a unified commitment to good health education and medical practices, by our government agencies, our medical community, and our citizenry that both doctors and patients can get on with the business of relieving pain and curing Lyme disease, thereby ensuring the continued leadership of the country.

As a parent and citizen, I am concerned about our beautiful landscaped park areas, particularly those near shopping and historic sites where families stroll leisurely and children play. I am concerned about school and community fields (usually bordered by woods and natural vegetation) where the children play soccer, field hockey, and football, fly kites or watch outdoor concerts and fireworks displays. These, in particular, are frequented by deer and birds and populated with ticks.

Although health departments—like many businesses today—are faced with budget cutbacks and increased responsibilities (such as protection from terrorism and potential biological threats), Lyme disease education and prevention should be considered one of those all-important priorities if we don't want our communities, states, and country to face a further economic and intellectual drain.

Max Planck, the Nobel Prize–winning German physicist credited with laying the groundwork for the development of the quantum theory, knew what it was like to fly in the face of established scientific thought. "A new scientific truth does not triumph by convincing its opponents and making them see the light," he said, "but rather because its opponents eventually die, and a new generation grows up that is familiar with it."

Thousands of men, women, and children with Lyme disease cannot wait for the greedy political foot-draggers to die before funding for research and treatment of this potent disease is made a priority. Too many of their own lives could be lost in the meantime.

Appendix A:
Glossary of Terms

acute phase A short, sharp, and relatively severe course of a disease; not chronic.

amino acid A family of modified organic acids that serve as building blocks for the synthesis of proteins.

amylase An enzyme that breaks down complex carbohydrates such as starch.

anorexia nervosa A personality disorder manifested by extreme aversion to food, usually occurring in young women.

antibiotics Drugs that work against bacteria.

antibodies Substances produced by the immune system to fight foreign invaders such as disease-causing microorganisms.

antidepressant Pharmaceutical agents used to treat clinical depression.

anti-inflammatories Agents that reduce inflammation without directly antagonizing the agent that caused it.

anxiety disorder Also known as anxiety neurosis or anxiety reaction, a condition that can be caused by psychological and physiological factors. It can take two general forms: (1) acute anxiety (panic disorder), marked by repeated occurrences of intense self-limited anxiety lasting usually a few minutes to an hour, or (2) chronic anxiety, characterized by less intense reactions of much longer duration (days, weeks, or months).

arthritis Inflammation of a joint.

autoimmune disease Disorders in which the body mounts a destructive immune response against its own tissues.

bacteria Microscopic germs that can cause infection.

Bell's palsy Partial facial paralysis due to inflammation around the facial nerve.

Borrelia A genus of bacteria with numerous species that cause disease in humans. The diseases associated with these organisms are typically relapsing conditions like Lyme disease.

Candida albicans A common saprophyte of the digestive tract and female urogenital tract. It does not ordinarily cause disease, but may do so following a disruption of bacterial flora of the body, or in patients with depressed immune systems.

case control study An epidemiological study that examines selected patients who have a defined disease (cases) with persons without the disease (controls).

case definition In the example of chronic fatigue syndrome (CFS), a combination of symptoms, signs, and physiological characteristics that serve to distinguish a case of CFS from other disease states.

Ceftin Trade name for the antibiotic cefuroxime axetil, approved by the FDA in 1996 for treatment of Lyme disease.

chronic Of long duration, denoting a disease of slow progress and long continuance.

Chronic Fatigue and Immune Dysfunction Syndrome (CFIDS) A synonym for chronic fatigue syndrome used by some patients and physicians.

coenzyme A substance that enhances or is necessary for the action of enzymes. These are generally much smaller than enzymes themselves.

co-morbid Two or more disease conditions that occur simultaneously within the same person.

connective tissue The supporting tissues of the body, such as tendons, ligaments, bone, and cartilage.

connective tissue disorder A variety of inflammatory diseases of connective tissue, the most common of which is rheumatoid arthritis. Much, if not all, of this disease is now attributed to autoimmune processes.

DEET A chemical insect repellent effective against ticks, for use on exposed skin.

delusional disorder A psychiatric disorder characterized by states of heightened self-awareness and a tendency toward paranoia.

dementia A biologically caused, permanent, progressive decline in intellectual function that interferes with the victim's normal social or economic activity.

depression A neurotic or psychotic condition marked by an inability to concentrate, insomnia, and feelings of dejection and guilt.

diuretic Agent that promotes the excretion of and/or increase in the amount of urine.

electrolyte Substance that dissociates in water to form a cation (positively charged ion) and anion (negatively charged ion). Charged ions are central to a variety of important processes in the body, including muscle contraction and nerve impulse conduction.

encephalitis Inflammation of the brain. Victims may experience confusion, irritability, spontaneous tearfulness, geographic disorientation, sleep disturbance, and impaired memory, attention, and/or verbal fluency.

encephalomyelitis Inflammation of the brain and spinal cord. Lyme encephalomyelitis may be mistakenly diagnosed as multiple sclerosis.

encephalopathy Disturbance or disease of the brain. In Lyme disease, this term usually refers to a patient who has developed cognitive problems.

enzyme Specialized protein that acts as catalyst for virtually all necessary chemical reactions that take place within the body. Like all catalysts, enzymes remain unchanged by the reactions they promote and will initiate many reactions until they are degraded (usually by another enzyme).

epidemic Outbreak of disease that affects a much greater number of people than is usual for the locality, or that spreads to regions where it is ordinarily not present.

epidemiology The branch of medical science that deals with the incidence, distribution, and control of disease in a population.

erythema migrans An expanding rash that is pathognomonic for Lyme disease, occurring shortly after the tick bite in many but not all patients. Satellite rashes may occur at later points in the illness. The most frequently mentioned "EM" is the bull's-eye, a red rash with central clearing that gradually enlarges. The EM rash may have a wide variety of other appearances as well.

etiology Causal association of a disease with an agent; the study of the cause of a disease.

false negative Test result indicating no disease when disease is actually present.

false positive Test result indicating disease when the disease in question is not present.

fibromyalgia A group of common rheumatoid disorders (not involving the joints) characterized by achy pain, tenderness, and stiffness of the muscles. Also known as myofascial pain syndrome and fibromyositis.

globulin A family of proteins found in abundance in plasma. Includes the gamma globulins, which in turn include the various antibody molecules produced by the immune system.

glucose A simple sugar, which is actively transferred into the blood, following the digestive breakdown of starch and other carbohydrates in the gut.

Herxheimer reaction This typically refers to an exacerbation of symptoms or new onset of symptoms shortly after starting antibiotic therapy due to a flaring of the immune system in response to the killing of the spirochetes.

idiopathic Denoting a disease of unknown cause.

imaging tests Any variety of methods for observing the internal anatomy of the body, ranging from simple X rays to complex three-dimensional scanning techniques using nuclear magnetic resonance, positron emission, and other techniques.

immune suppressants Agents that block or restrict the activity of one or more components of the immune system, usually leading to the increased susceptibility to infectious disease.

insomnia Inability to sleep even in the absence of external impediments, during the period when sleep should normally occur.

Lyme carditis Result of the presence of live organisms in the heart; cardiac manifestations typically begin 1–2 months after the initial infection (ranging from 1 week to 7 months) and may occur as an isolated event or coincidental with other complaints.

lymph nodes Secondary organs throughout the body that play a central role in the activation and trafficking of immune lymphocytes in the body.

Magnetic Resonance Imaging (MRI) The use of nuclear magnetic resonance of protons to produce cross-sectional proton density images of internal structures of the human body.

malabsorption syndrome Results from impaired absorption of nutrients from the bowel.

malaise A feeling of general discomfort or uneasiness, an out-of-sorts feeling, often the first indication of an infection or other disease.

meningitis Inflammation of the meninges surrounding the brain. Patients may experience headache, light sensitivity, and pain when moving head, nausea and vomiting. Patients with Lyme disease typically develop this as an early neurologic reaction to Lyme infection.

multiple chemical sensitivity disorder A controversial diagnosis of an allergy-like sensitivity to an unusually broad range and number of substances. This condition has not been subjected to rigorous scientific scrutiny, and there is considerable doubt as to whether it actually exists.

multiple sclerosis A slowly progressive central nervous system disease characterized by disseminated patches of demyelination in the brain and spinal cord.

myalgic encephalomyelitis A synonym for chronic fatigue syndrome in common usage in the United Kingdom and Canada.

myoglobin The oxygen-transporting protein of muscle, resembling blood hemoglobin in function.

narcolepsy A sudden, uncontrollable disposition to sleep occurring at irregular intervals with or without obvious predisposing or exciting cause.

neuromyasthenia Muscular weakness, usually of emotional origin.

neuropsychiatric Relating to organic and functional diseases of the nervous system.

neuropsychological testing A formal battery of tests of brain functions, such as auditory and visual memory, auditory and visual attention, visual motor performance, intelligence, speed of mental processing, verbal fluency, and mental flexibility.

neurotransmitter Substance produced in neurons that promote or inhibit the conduction of nerve impulses such as epinephrine, norepinephrine, dopamine, serotonin, and gamma-amniobutyrate.

nymph Immature stage of a tick's life cycle, between larval and adult, when transmission of Lyme disease to humans is most likely to occur.

pathognomonic Characteristic or indicative of a disease denoting especially one or more typical symptoms.

pathophysiology Derangement of function caused by disease.

permethrin An insecticide effective against ticks, for use on clothing but not the skin.

Polymerase Chain Reaction (PCR) One of the tests used to help detect the genetic material of the spirochete that causes Lyme disease.

Positron Emission Tomography (PET scan) Imaging technique that relies on the detection of gamma rays emitted from tissues after administration of a natural biochemical substance into which positron-emitting isotopes have been incorporated.

pulmonary Relating to the lungs.

radiculopathy A disturbance in the nerve that may cause shooting pain, numbness, or tingling in the distribution of nerve root. Emanates from the spinal cord.

renal Relating to the kidneys.

schizophrenia A group of psychotic disorders characterized by extensive withdrawal from reality, illogical thinking patterns, delusions, and hallucinations and accompanied by other emotional and behavioral disturbances.

sequelae Morbid conditions as a consequence of a disease.

seronegative or seropositive titers Blood tests indicating either a negative or positive reaction to antibodies for Lyme.

Single Photon Emission Computed Tomography (SPECT scan) An imaging technique that measures the emission of photons of a given energy from radioactive tracers introduced into the body. As with other forms of computer-assisted tomography, the technique produces a series of cross-sectional images of internal anatomy.

spirochete A type of bacteria with a slender spiral shape.

subacute A zone between acute and chronic, denoting the course of the disease.

systemic lupus erythematosus An inflammatory disease of connective tissue occurring predominately in women (90 percent). It is considered to be an autoimmune disease.

titer The concentration of a substance in a solution or the strength of such a substance detected by titration. The term is most likely to refer to antibody titer, which is a measure of the concentration of specific antibodies to selected microbes that are circulating in an individual's bloodstream.

vasculitis Inflammation of the blood vessels. Many diseases can cause vasculitis, such as lupus, syphilis, Lyme disease, and primary angiitis of the central nervous system.

vitamin A group of organic micronutrients, present in minute quantities in natural foodstuffs that are essential to normal metabolism.

Appendix B:
Lyme Disease Support Groups (LDSG)*

ALABAMA
LDSG of Alabama
Julianne Collins
1736 15th Avenue South
Birmingham, AL 35205
205-281-1248

LDSG of Alabama—Central
  Chapter
Jim Schmidt
1852 Country Road 57
Prattville, AL 36067
334-358-3206
E-mail: jschm47974@aol.com

LDSG of Alabama—North
  Chapter
Carol Potts and Kara Tyson
2070 Schillinger Road South
Mobile, AL 36695
256-539-3033

LDSG of Alabama—South
  Chapter
Les Roberts
850-478-5270

ALASKA
Alaska Military Lyme Support
Colleen Nicholson
18909 Sarichef Loop
Eagle River, AK 99577
907-622-3244
E-mail: jcn4jc@aol.com

ARIZONA
Arizona LDSG
Carol Marter
1821 North 87th Way
Scottsdale, AZ 85257
480-994-5449
E-mail: CarolM94@aol.com or
Lisa Katz
8432 East Lincoln Drive
Scottsdale, AZ 85250

*Courtesy of the Lyme Disease Association and The Lyme Alliance

ARKANSAS
Fairfield Bay Lyme SG
Mary Alice Beer
112 Hollybrook Road
Fairfield Bay, AR 72088
501-884-3502

CALIFORNIA
Advocates 4 health: Tick-borne
  Disease SHG
Sheryl Glidden
Advocates of Zoonotic Disease
  Awareness
c/o PALS, P.O. Box 1271
San Luis Obispo, CA 93406
805-544-0984
E-mail: advocates4health
  @yahoo.com

Butte County LDSG
Sue Caldwell
6712 Chapman Lane
Paradise, CA 95969
530-877-0623 or
Marlene Hauck
7664 Citrus Avenue
Oroville, CA 95966
530-877-0623
E-mail: mar@cncnet.com

Danvers/East Bay LDSG
Carol Martin
341 Bolero Drive
Danville, CA 94526
E-mail: sarajohn1@mindspring.
  com

LDSG of San Diego County
Nancy Seppala
8115 Whitehead Place
La Mesa, CA 91942
619-596-4963
E-mail: NancySEPP@aol.com

Los Angeles LDSG
Barbara Hunt
Monrovia, California
E-mail: canynbugbarb@aol.com
Website: http://hometown.aol.com/
  canynbugbarb/myhomepage/
  collection.html

Lyme Disease Resource Center
Phyllis Mervine
P.O. Box 1423
Ukiah, CA 95482

Marin Lyme Disease Support
  Group
Lee Lull
103 Walnut Avenue
Corte Madera, CA 94925
415-927-9553
E-mail: leema@earthlink.net

Mid-Peninsula LDSG
Karen Chew
1025 Williams Way #3
Mountain View, CA 94040
800-216-5556
E-mail: ldsg_karren@hotmail.
  com or

El Camino Hospital
2500 Grant Road, Room D
Mountain View, CA 94040
800-216-5556
E-mail: abfromca@hotmail.com

Monterey County Lyme SG
Patrizia Ahlers-Johnson
19145 Mallory Canyon Road
Salinas, CA 93907

NorCaLymers
Darcie E. Little
San Jose, California
E-mail: NorCaLymers-owner
  @yahoogroups.com or
  daliddle1@aol.com
Website: http://groups.yahoo.
  com/group/NorCaLymers

North Central CA LDSG
Laura Lee Ames
325 Fresno Street
Coalinga, CA 93210

North Coast LDSG
Jentri Anders, Ph.D.
3883 Patricks Point Drive,
  Space 12
Trinidad, CA 95570
E-mail: jentri@tidepool.com

Orange and L.A. Counties LDSG
Earis Corman
13904F Rio Hondo Circle
La Mirada, CA 90638
E-mail: eariscorman@aol.com

San Francisco LDSG
Elisabeth Feldman
San Francisco, California
415-273-5833
Use e-mail
E-mail: elsbeth@pacbell.net

Santa Cruz LDSG
Sarah Weiss
Aptos, California
831-662-3628
Use e-mail
E-mail: AramSarah@cs.com
Website: www.angelfire.com/
  punky/lymedisease/index.html

Seacoast LDSG
Charise Ott
5561 Ludlow Avenue
Garden Grove, CA 92845

Sierra Foothills Lyme Support
Meg Hughes and Peggy
  Leonardo
16713 Hillaire Road
Rough & Ready, CA 95975
530-432-4280 or 530-272-3204
E-mail: Hughes@news.com

Siskyou County LDSG and
  National Teenage Network
Solitaire Metheny
Montague, California
530-459-5571
E-mail for information
E-mail: Solitaire@snowcrest.net

Sonoma Valley Hospital LDSG
Sonoma Valley
Brent Sieloff
Phone for information
707-833-6296

Sonoma Valley LDSG
Thora Graves
105 Wisteria Circle
Cloverdale, CA 95425

South Central CA LDSG
Laura Lee Ames
325 Fresno Street
Coalinga, CA 93210

Southcoast LDSG
Mark LaFevers
7028 Shepard Mesa Drive
Carpenteria, CA 93013

Southern California LDSG
Joy DeMeta
Lake Elsinore, California
909-674-0455
E-mail for information
E-mail: Joy@aJoy2cre8.com

Ticked-Off
Laura Lee Ames
325 Fresno Street
Coalinga, CA 93210

Trinity County LD Network
Nancy Brown or Elizabeth
   Halterman

P.O. Box 707
Weaverville, CA 96093
530-623-3227 or 530-623-4795
E-mail: lnbrown@snowcrest.net

CONNECTICUT
Fairfield County LDSG
Maureen Albertson
42 Broadbridge Road
Bridgeport, CT 06610
203-374-3844

Friends of the Easton Library
Dolly Curtis
35 Flat Rock Road
Easton, CT 06612

Greater Danbury LDSG
Pat Bartlett
41 Church Hill Road
Redding, CT 06896
E-mail: PIBINQUIRE@aol.com

Greater Hartford LDS and
   Action Committee
Chris Montes
139 Perry Street
Unionville, CT 06085 or
Randy Sykes
5 Lost Brook Road
West Simsbury, CT 06092

Greenwich LDSG
Jody Ring
P.O. Box 31269
Greenwich, CT 06831

Lyme Disease Coalition of
 NY/ CT
Barbara Goldklang
P.O. Box 463
Katonah, NY 10536
914-769-6243

Lyme Disease Network of
 Connecticut
Cynthia Herms, M.S.W.
8 Pamela Court
Broad Brook, CT 06016

Newton Task Force
Maggie Shaw
82 Eden Hill Road
Newton, CT 06470

Ridgefield Lyme Disease Task
 Force
Karen Gaudian
29 Woodland Way
Ridgefield, CT 06877

SECT Chronic LSG
Kathleen Dickson and
 Judi Karol
Waterford, Connecticut
Phone for information
860-599-5451 or 860-437-9865

Ticked Off Lyme
Steven Gottschalk
2490 Black Rock Turnpike
 #327
Fairfield, CT 06432

Time For Lyme, Inc.
Diane Blanchard
48 Londonderry Drive
New Greenwich, CT 06830 or
Debbie Siciliano
19 Lower Cross Road
Greenwich, CT 06831
Website: www.TimeForLyme.
 org

TRISHA (Tick-Related Illness SH
 Alliance)
Nancy Berntsen
6 West Street
Columbia, CT 06237
860-228-5087
E-mail: trisha@oikourgos.
 com
Website: http://www.oikourgos.
 com/trisha

Wilton Lyme Disease Support
 Group
Allison Clark
30 Howell Tree Place
Wilton, CT 06897 or
Douglas Bunnell, Ph.D.
436 Danbury Road
Wilton, CT 06897
203-834-1635
E-mail: BDCZ@aol.com

Wilton Area LDSG for Teens and
 Kids
Merry Frons
E-mail: mfrons@aol.com

DELAWARE
Delaware Lyme SG
Susan Driver
4926 Old Capitol Trail
Wilmington, DE 19808
302-996-9065
E-mail: Tlizzy@snip.net

FLORIDA
Cat Hospital of Orlando
M. Alexandra Stowe, D.V.M.
266 East Altamonte Drive
Altamonte Springs, FL 32701

Eye on Lyme Network
Maria Granda—Rehabilitation
  Counselor
2709 Art Museum Drive
Jacksonville, FL 32207
904-535-1120

Florida Lyme Association
Fred Lawson
5029 El Destino Drive
Leesburg, FL 34748
352-360-2301
E-mail: flalyme@handtechisp.
  com

Florida Lyme Disease Network
Marvina Lodge, President
4166 Oak Grove Drive
Zellwood, FL 32798
407-880-LYME (5963)
E-mail: loveyonlyme@aol.
  com

Website: www.groups.yahoo.
  com/group/LoveyOnLyme

LSG of North Florida
Richard A. Goldman,
  D.V.M.
4209 NW 37th Place
Gainesville, FL 32606
352-373-8055

Suncoast Lyme Support
  Network
Marilyn Kerr, R.N.
5100 Burchette Road #1003
Tampa, FL 33647
813-977-0629
E-mail: marilynk@tampabay.
  rr.com
Website: http://web.tampabay.
  rr.com/lymecfs/suncoast/html

GEORGIA
Georgia Lyme Disease
  Association
Diane McCoy
2061 Ursuline Way Northwest
Acworth, GA 30101 or
Marilyn Steinbach
3350 Pebble Hill Drive
Marietta, GA 30062
678-560-7496
E-mail: Mstein47@aol.com or
Lance Brubaker
678-473-9643
E-mail: lyme@attbi.com

ILLINOIS
Chicagoland LDSG
Lisa Winkates or
  Kim Drescher
Eisenhower Public Library
4652 North Olcott
Harwood Heights, IL 60706
E-mail: mercuryspice@aol.com
  or Liebekim@mediaone.net
Website: http://www.hometown.
  aol.com/mercuryspice/
  myhomepageindex.html

East Central Illinois LDS
Susanna Rose Warner
902 West William Street
Champaign, IL 61821

Illowa Lyme Disease
  Network
Lillian Hensley or Marilyn
  McBride
P.O. Box 10
Reynolds, IL 61279
309-799-5500 or
  309-372-4472
E-mail: CVKEITH@aol.com or
  marilynmcb@mcics.com

Mississippi Valley LD
  Network
Lou Ellen Gooding
P.O. Box 568
Roseville, IL 61473
309-426-2339
E-mail: louellen@midwest.net

Northern Illinois Lyme
  Resources
Jeanette Wheat
Batavia, IL 60510
630-406-0393
E-mail: Ggrom48@aol.com
Website: http://members.
  aol.com/nilr/LYME.
  HTM

Southern Illinois LSG
Katherine Godell
1211 West Hill Avenue
Carbondale, IL 62901
618-549-1775
E-mail: tgodell@siu.edu

INDIANA
Central Indiana LDSG
Theresa Parks
3152 Thayer Street
Indianapolis, IN 46222
317-297-1695

NW Indiana Lyme
  Education, Awareness,
  and Prevention
Jeri Wright
722 Baums Bridge Road
Kouts, IN 46347
219-766-3068
E-mail: lymieinin@
  hotmail.com
Website: www.expage.
  com/lymeinfoinnwin

Terre Haute LDSG
Connie Lawrence
7122 Rosedale Road
Terre Haute, IN 47805
812-466-1469

Vanderburgh County LDSG
Charlene Glover
Evansville, Illinois
812-471-1990

IOWA
Iowa Lyme Disease Association
Cathy Cuddeback
P.O. Box 291
Brighton, IA 52540
319-698-2013
E-mail: mstarfarm@se-iowa.net
Website: www.
   iowalymediseaseassoc.com

Iowa LDA, Ames Chapter
Geri Fosseen or Judy Wegg
Route 2
Radcliffe, IA 50230
319-698-2013

Iowa LDA, Coralville Chapter
LaDonna Wicklund
1826 Brown Deer Cove
Coralville, IA 52241

Iowa LDA, Mason City
   Chapter
Tammi Poppe
515-357-8037

Iowa LDA, Scott City Chapter
Kris Woodward
2326 Scott Street
Davenport, IA 52803

Quad-Cities LD Network
Marilyn McBride
4025 Aspen Hills Drive
Bettendorf, IA 52722
319-332-7660

KANSAS
Lyme Association of Greater
   Kansas City (Kansas and
   Missouri)
Ed Olson
P.O. Box 25853
Overland Park, KS 66225 or
Mary McCutchan
P.O. Box 6704
Leawood, KS 66206
Lyme Hot Line:
   913-438-LYME (5963)
E-mail: lymefight@aol.com

Lyme Link in Lawrence
Steve and Carol Grieb
2509 Stowe Drive
Lawrence, KS 66049
E-mail: dagriebs@aol.com

KENTUCKY
Northern Kentucky Tri-State
   Lyme-Vine SG
Candace Young
606-283-1038

MAINE
Eastern Maine LDSG
Happy Dickey
132 Main Road South
Hampden, ME 04444 or
Tim Worster
207-884-7914
E-mail: TimWor12
  @netscape.net

MARYLAND
After the Bite
Lucy Barnes
P.O. Box 232
Church Hill, MD 21623

Central Maryland LDSG
Richard Poole
2956 Old Taneytown Road
Westminster, MD 21158 or
Robin Ann and Jay Wolfenden
113 Bertie Avenue
Westminster, MD 21157

Harford County LDSG
Jean Galbreath
P.O. Box 13
Street, MD 21154
410-838-LYME (5963)
E-mail: lyme@starix.net

LDA of the Eastern Shore
Jackie King
8745 Williams Mill Pond
  Road
Delmar, MD 21875

Mid-Atlantic LD Resource
  Center, L.L.C.
M. David and Marsha LeBrun
15701 Yeoho Road
Sparks, MD 21152

Owings Mills LDSG
Scott and Billi Jo Kirk
506 Granleigh Road
Owings Mills, MD 21117
E-mail: bjkirk@home.com

Woodbine LDSG
Cathy Fleishman
2170 State Road 94
Woodbine, MD 21797

MASSACHUSETTS
Boston Lyme Disease Resource
  Line
Kerry Kineavy, R.N.
843 East 2nd Street
South Boston, MA 02127
617-268-3767

Burlington LDSG
Gloria Stone
45 Cresthaven Drive
Burlington, MA 01803
781-272-9786
E-mail: grandmaglo@cs.com

Central Massachusetts LD
  Family Help Line
Eileen Johnson
Webster, Massachusetts

Phone for information
508-943-2692

Greater Boston LD Resource
    Center
Dan Ardrey
Brookline, Massachusetts
617-739-1498

Islington LDSG
Westwood Public Library,
    Islington Branch
280 Washington Street, Route 1A
Islington, MA 02090
E-mail: linhillymema@aol.com

LDA, Cape Cod Chapter
Karen Hallett-LaRoche
18 Cedric Drive
Centerville, MA 02632 or
Terri Reiser
1146 Route 134, #4C
S. Dennis, MA 02660

LD Awareness Assoc. of Western
    Massachusetts
Marci Linker
P.O. Box 60604
Florence, MA 01062

LD Self-Help and Information
    Group of North Central
    Massachusetts
Dawn Paradis
163 Barker Hill Road

Townsend, MA 01469
978-597-2726
E-mail: dgipa@yahoo.com

Lower Cape LDSG
Diane Heart or Marci Rose
1145 Main Street
Brewster, MA 02631
508-896-6189 or 508-292-9237

LymeLight Suport Group
Rae Record
36 James Circle
Mashpee, MA 02649

Mansfield Lyme Disease
    Resource Center
Gail Beers
30 Beaumont Pond Road
Mansfield, MA 02048
508-261-0230

Massachusetts LD Coalition
John Coughlan
P.O. Box 1916
Mashpee, MA 02649
508-563-7033

Middlesex County LD Self-Help
    and Information Group
Linda Hilliard, R.N., C.R.N.A.
20 D-1 Rainbow Pond Drive
Walpole, MA 02081
866-596-3435 (toll-free)
Website: www.lymehelp.org

New Bedford Lyme Support
Friends
Denise Chasse
New Bedford, Massachusetts
508-979-7859

North Shore LD Information
and SG
Kay Lyon
49 Porter Street
Wenham, MA 01984
978-468-6336
E-mail: b10g7@mediaone.net

Outer Cape LDSG
Carolyn Tacke
Truro, Massachusetts
508-487-2720

Plymouth LDSG
Janet Stroup
11 Plymouth
Carver, MA 02330
508-866-9476
E-mail: LDSGofPlymouth@
aol.com

South Shore LD Resource Line
Dominique Baytarian
26 Fox Hill Circle
Marshfield, MA 02330
781-837-5342

Upper Cape LDSG
Carolyn Ashbaugh

27 Little Island Road
Falmouth, MA 02540

Western Massachusetts LD
Resource Line
Sue Schribner and Marci Linker
Florence, Massachusetts
413-247-5884
E-mail: Woodi16@aol.com

Westport/Fall River LSDG
Polly Emilitas, Janice Dey,
Beth Herosy
795 Pine Hill Road
Westport, MA 02790
508-636-3184

Westwood LD Resource
Line
Maureen O'Brien, R.N.
71 Cedar Lane
Westwood, MA 02090
781-251-2521

MICHIGAN
Clio LDSG
Clarice Engelheart
3373 East Vienna
Clio, MI 48420

Flint Area LDSG
Mary Fairweather
3373 East Vienna
Clio, MI 48420
810-686-9383

Ironwood LSG
Peg Sutherland
North 10561 Grand View Lane
Ironwood, MI 49938

Jackson, Hillsdale, and
    Calhoun Co. LDSG
Sharon Smith
12235 Folks Road
Hanover, MI 49241

Kalamazoo LSG
Natalie Escandon
7889 North 40th Street
Augusta, MI 49012
616-731-2031

Ludington Phone Support
Terry Hermann
616-845-7704

LDA of Ann Arbor
Dr. Neal and Meredith Spencer
    Foster
2115 Georgetown Boulevard
Ann Arbor, MI 48105
734-663-0756
E-mail: nealfost@umich.
    edu

Lyme Alliance, Inc.
Sharon Smith
P.O. Box 454
Concord, MI 49237
E-mail: barbfitz@chartermi.
    net

Mid-Michigan Support Group
Grace Lutheran Church
Saginaw, Michigan
888-784-5963

North Oakland County
Carol Fisch
248-625-5275
E-mail: EJFisch@aol.com

Oakland/ Malcomb/ St.Clair
    County LDSG
Linda Lobes; Troy Library
888-784-LYME (5963)
E-mail: Lpurdy1040@
    aol.com

Wayne County LDSG
Connie Siese
35431 Brush Street
Wayne, MI 48184
734-326-3502
E-mail: CSLYME@aol.com

MINNESOTA
Cloquet Support Group
Lannei Lammi and
    Sandy Karpinen
115 St. Louis Avenue
Cloquet, MN 55720
218-879-9968

Lyme Disease Coalition of
    Minnesota
Lynn Olivier
1613 Hewitt Avenue

St. Paul, MN 55104
651-644-7239
E-mail: lymenet_mn
  @yahoo.com

LymeNet North Metro SG
Lynn Olivier
1613 Hewitt Avenue
St. Paul, MN 55104
651-644-7239
E-mail: lynnolivier@bigfoot.com

Mid-State Minnesota
  LDSG
Geoffrey Steiner
24229 Basswood Road
Cushing, MN 56443

Minnesota Lyme Disease
  Coalition
Tom Grier
902 Grandview Avenue
Duluth, MN 55812
218-728-3914

Thief River Falls LDSG
Kathy and Andy Mehrkens
10992 140 Avenue Northwest
Thief River Falls, MN 56704

We Care Lyme Disease
  Support Group
Pearl Brennan
1916 NE 4th Avenue
Austin, MN 55912
507-433-6400

Wilmar Lyme Support Group
Lynn Zimmer
14250 90th Street Southwest
Raymond, MN 56282
320-967-4306

MISSISSIPPI
LDSG of Mississippi
Linda Beasley
1540 Adams Lake Road
Utica, MS 39175
601-855-2064
E-mail: LKBeasley@
  aol.com

MISSOURI
Green Hills LDSG
Suzanne Coulter
900 Jefferson Street
Chillicothe, MO 64601

Lyme Association of Greater
  Kansas City (Kansas and
  Missouri)
Carol Grieb
P.O. Box 6704
Leawood, KS 66206
Lyme Hot Line: 913-Get-Lyme
  (438-5963)
E-mail: lymefight@aol.com
Website: www.community.
  lawrence.com/info/
  LymeAssociation

SW Missouri LDSG
Marol Jean Royer

241 Journey Drive
Mashfield, MO 65700

NEBRASKA
Midwest Alliance for
  Understanding LD
Mary Gentry
5051 Road 197
Lewellen, NE 69147

NEVADA
Visiting Physician Program—
  Las Vegas
Rene Landis, Coordinator
2712 St. Clair Drive
Las Vegas, NV 89128
702-256-9776
E-mail: Reeeneee@aol.com

NEW HAMPSHIRE
New Hampshire LDSG
Mary Fanslau
R.R. 1 Box 15
Strafford, NH 03884

NEW JERSEY
Cape May County LDSG
Edina Gibb
Cape May, New Jersey
609-463-8411
E-mail: edina@uscom.com

Greater Raritan LDSG
Jeannine Der Bedrosian
13 Thomas Road
East Brunswick, NJ 08816

Hunterdon County LDSG
Sarah Melvin
P.O. Box 161
Little York, NJ 08834

LD Information Group of
  Burlington City
Sue Huesken
P.O. Box 41
Palmyra, NJ 08065
856-461-3369
E-mail: sueted@
  bellatlantic.net

Lehigh Lyme League
Betty DiDario
50 Puddingstone Way
Phillipsburg, NJ 08868

Long Valley LDSG
Nancy Braithewaite
6 Lenore Court
Long Valley, NJ 07853 or
Helen Fasy
2 Sparrow Lane
Long Valley, NJ 07853
908-813-1134
E-mail: liveitup@eclipse.net

Lyme Care SG
Judy Debow
Wrightstown, New Jersey
609-758-9155

Lyme Disease Web Page
Joe Burke

3 Braxton Way
Glassboro, NJ 08028

Lymelight LDSG
Jane Chapman
83 Glasglow Road
Williamstown, NJ 08094
609-629-2446

Lyme Vaccine Victims
Jenny Mara, R.N.
1308 Turner Avenue
Ocean, NJ 07712

Mandy Memorial LDSG
Mary Schmidt
42 Elizabeth Street
Sayerville, NJ 08872
732-238-6405

Morris County LSG
Jennifer Krasinski
300 Morris Avenue
Mountain Lakes, NJ 07046 or
Reid McMurray
42 Fox Hill Road
Denville, NJ 07834
973-627-0345
E-mail: rcmcmur3194@aol.com

NJ Tick Talk
Donna Robertson
P.O. Box 65
Leeds Point, NJ 08220
856-461-3369
E-mail: TickTalkNJ@aol.com

North Jersey LDSG
Jeffery Simons
276 Indian Trail Drive
Franklin Lakes, NJ 07417

Somerville Medical
  Center LSG
Sharon Eaton
110 Rehill Avenue
Somerville, NJ 08876
908-685-2814

Sussex County Lyme Group
Tim Rowett and Evelyn Teri
28 Glenwood Mountain Road
Sussex, NJ 07461
973-875-6842

NEW MEXICO
Lyme Disease Action Network
Jan Borra
3417 Morningside Drive
  Northeast
Albuquerque, NM 87110

NEW YORK
Albany LDSG
Stephanie Bayan
28-36 Burt Street
Ft. Edward, NY 12828

Hudson Valley LD
  Committee
Jill Auerbach
143 Bart Drive
Poughkeepsie, NY 12603

Hyde Park LDSG
Claire Nuttall
94 Roosevelt Road
Hyde Park, NY 12538

LDA of Queens
Norman Rosenthal
81-19 Lefferts Boulevard
Kew Gardens, NY 11415

LD Coalition of New York
    and Connecticut
Barbara Goldklang
P.O. Box 463
Katonah, NY 10536
914-769-6243

LDSG of Brooklyn and Staten
    Island
Thomas and Janet Jemec
1 Ebony Court
Brooklyn, NY 11229
E-mail: pumpkin501@aol.com
    or Janjem1@aol.com

Long Island LDSG
Bob Levine
Long Island, New York
516-473-4389
E-mail: omicron@erols.com

Long Island Lyme Association
Diane Leary
P.O. Box 1842
North Massapequa, NY 11758
516-893-LYME (5963)

Lyme Borrelia Outreach
    Foundation
Stephan J. Nostrom, R.N.
P.O. Box 496
Mattituck, NY 11952
516-298-9606

Mid-Hudson LDSG
Rachel Dildilian
27 Mill Road
Hyde Park, NY 12538

Mid-Westchester LDSG
Suzanne Sugar
6 Southview Road
Chappaqua, NY 10514
914-238-8801

New York City LDSG
Ellen Lubarsky
315 West 86th Street,
    Apt. 2E
New York, NY 10024

No. Dutchess LDSG
Mary Belliveau
No. Dutchess Bible Church
Fisk Street
Red Hook, NY 12571

Northport Lyme Disease
    Ed/SG
Judi Hason
Northport Library
1515 Laurel Avenue
Northport, NY 11768

Rockland County LDSG
Rushana White
60 Tranquillity Road
Suffern, NY 10901 or
Sandy Mellion
7 Hickory Lane
New City, NY 10965

Southern Dutchess LDSG
Pat Baldt
19 Gerald Drive, Apt. E3
Poughkeepsie, NY 12601

Suffolk County LSG
Bob Levine
201 Washington Avenue
Port Jefferson, NY 11777

Westchester Children's
   LDSG
Barbara Goldklang
35 Old Farm Road South
Pleasantville, NY 10570

Westchester LDSG
Mark Kramer
P.O. Box 82
Irvington, NY 10533

NORTH CAROLINA
North Carolina Lyme Disease
   Foundation, Inc.
Elizabeth Jordan, D.V.M.
7405 Louisburg Road
Raleigh, NC 27616

NORTH DAKOTA
Minot LDSG
Lloyd Ann Caston
1810 66th Street
   Northwest
Minot, ND 58703

OHIO
Columbus Lyme Support
Alice Stacy
4784 Valley Forge Drive
Columbus, OH 43229
614-888-4392

Dayton LDSG
Sharon Davis and Linda Flory,
   L.P.N.
Dayton, Ohio
513-932-5475 or
   973-885-7880

Greater Cleveland LDSG
Ann Hirschberg
7644 Main Street
Cleveland, OH 44138
440-235-4163
E-mail: gcldsg
   @aol.com
Website: www.geocities.com/
   gcldsg

LDA of Ohio
Carol Long
601 Daventry Lane
Gahanna, OH 43230

Mahoney LDSG
Marge Helle
2904 Julian Street
Youngstown, OH 44502

Mansfield LDS
Jim Zara
626 Koogle Road
Mansfield, OH 44903
419-589-5622

Marietta Lyme Support
Becky Madine, R.N.
Marietta, Ohio
614-374-6971

Toledo Lyme Support
Sue Umphress
Toledo, Ohio
419-634-6596

Tri-State LDSG
Linda Von Hoene
5815 Bramble Avenue
Cincinnati, OH 45227
513-561-5794

Warrant County LSG
Linda Flory
9931 Bunnell Hill Road
Centerville, OH 45458
937-885-7880

OREGON
Northwest Lyme Disease Network
Vicki Lawson

5510 Highway 30 West
The Dalles, OR 97058
541-296-9597
E-mail: vicki@gorge.net

Northwest Lyme Disease Support
   Network
Rita Stanley, Ph.D.
7740 SW Miner Way
Portland, OR 97225
503-413-7348
E-mail: ritastan@worldnet.
   att.net

Oregon Lyme Disease Network
Theresa Denham
24780 Dodds Road
Bend, OR 97701

PENNSYLVANIA
Central Bucks LSG
Susan MacNamee, Camille
   Wieder
215-529-9456
E-mail: aqua920@aol.com

Central PA LDSG
Luke Glick
R.R. 5
Selinsgrove, PA 17870 or
Patty Smith
570-275-4464
E-mail: haroldsm@sunlink.net

Doylestown LSG
Susan MacNamee

1123 Dublin Pike
Perkasie, PA 18944 or
Sue Onraet
116 Hampshire Drive
Chalfont, PA 18914

Elk County LSG
Yoland and Joe Wofel
458 Wofel Avenue
St. Mary's, PA 15857

Gettysburg PA LDSG
Vickie Karam Smith
1933 Biglerville Road
Gettysburg, PA 17325 or
Lovette Mott
2389 Chambersburg Road
Biglerville, PA 17307

Grove City LD Information
   SG
Lisa Robinson
98 Whittaker School Road
Grove City, PA 16127
724-458-0509

LDA of Southeast Pennsylvania
Harvey Kliman, Ph.D.
P.O. Box 944
Chadds Ford, PA 19317

LDSG for South Central
   Pennsylvania
Dave Nelson
354 Maple Street
Columbia, PA 17512

Lehigh Valley LDSG
Michelle Gass
534 Diamond Street
Slatington, PA 18080 or
Michelle Raber and Camille
   Wieder
31 Belmont Avenue Rear
Quakertown, PA 18951
610-767-7964 or
   215-529-9456
E-mail: symphony@enter.
   net

LSG of Erie County
Deborah Abbot
3661 Hershey Road
Erie, PA 16506

LYMECURE
Joel Shmukler, Esquire
105 Cheswold Court
Wayne, PA 19087
610-947-2058
E-mail: jmspaesg@aol.com or
   LYMECURE@aol.com

Lyme Disease Community
   Coalition
Stephen Cohen
P.O. Box 236
Downingtown, PA 19355 or
401 Baker Lane
Coatsville, Pennsylvania
610-384-9622
E-mail: LYME911@
   aol.com

Mensa Lyme LDSG
David Bartholomew
323 Chapel Avenue
Allentown, PA 18103

New Hope LSG of
   Quarryville
Nadine Lingo
New Hope Office
215 W. 4th Street, Suite 107
Quarryville, PA 17566
717-786-2802
E-mail: Dufalo@aol.com

Northwest Pennsylvania
   LDSG
David and Sally Coates
R.R. 4 Box 342
Sugar Grove, PA 16350

Pediatric Lyme Disease
   Association
Terry Vosburgh
P.O. Box 381
Unionville, PA 19375

Quarryville LDSG
Ken Zieber
215 West 4th Street,
   Suite 105
Quarryville, PA 17566

Pittsburgh South Hills LDSG
Tammy Burleson-Berkoben
1805 Hankins Drive
McKeesport, PA 15135

Southern Tier Lyme
Marianne Sheppeck
205 No. Pennsylvania Avenue
Sayre, PA 18840

Western PA Lyme Information
Ronda Bartholomew
6986 East State Street
Hermitage, PA 16148

RHODE ISLAND
LDSG of Rhode Island
Richard Desrosiers
Warwick Central Public
   Library
600 Sandy Lane
Warwick, RI 02889
401-392-1262
E-mail: RhodeIslandLyme
   @yahoo.com or
   sbrand@efortress.com

LDA, Rhode Island Chapter
Lisa Larisa
77 Argyle Avenue
East Providence, RI 02915 or
Julie E. Meolla
132 Windermere Way
Warwick, RI 02886 or
Lore Gray
3 Otan Court
East Greenwich, RI 02818

Newport County Lyme Disease
   Support Group
Richard LaFerriere

24 Vernon Avenue
Newport, RI 02840
401-847-2657
E-mail: marennes
  @compuserve.com

Rhode Island LDSG
Janet Cooper
53 Conanicus Avenue, Unit 3B
Jamestown, RI 02835
E-mail: duke@jamestownri.
  com

Westport/ Fall River LDSG
Janice Dey
69 Cliff Street
Tiverton, RI 02878 or
Beth Herosy
Feng Shui Center
269 South Main Street
Providence, RI 02903

SOUTH CAROLINA
Lyme Disease Network of South
  Carolina
Sue Fox
209 Argyll Road
Columbia, SC 29212

SOUTH DAKOTA
South Dakota Lyme Support
Penny Sue Story
27116 Bluebird Place
Harrisburg, SD 57032
605-743-2071
E-mail: lpstory@aol.com

TENNESSEE
LD Network of Middle Tennessee
Bonnie Huntsinger
7700 Indian Springs Drive
Nashville, TN 37221

Mid-South Lyme Disease SG
Cheryl Leventhal
5336 Mason Road
Memphis, TN 38120
901-682-3188

Nashville LDSG
Green Hills Branch Library
3701 Benham Avenue
Nashville, TN 37215
E-mail: lyme@comcast.net

TEXAS
Lyme Disease Network, Texas
Brenda Pitts
701 Meadowdale Drive
Royse City, TX 75189
E-mail: BPB123@
  earthlink.net

Northwest Houston Lyme
  Support Group
Teresa Lucher
18110 Glenledi Drive
Houston, TX 77084
E-mail: Teresag143@aol.
  com or
K. Blanco
E-mail: snakecharmer_s
  @yahoo.com

Texas Lyme Coalition
Lisa Johnson
2001 Blue Sage Drive
Cedar Park, TX 78613
E-mail: lisa@txlyme.org
Website: www.txlyme.org

Texas Lyme Support Group
Karla Pollock
2 Edgehill Road
Joshua, TX 76058

UTAH
Mountain West Lyme Disease
  Support Group
Shelly Wolf
226 Daniel Drive
Tooele, UT 84074

VERMONT
Partners in Lyme
Amy Kelley
12 Hitzel Terrace
Rutland, VT 05701

VIRGINIA
Central Virginia
  LDSG
Pat Arnold
P.O. Box 567
Gordonville, VA 22942
540-832-2903

Lyme Association of Virginia, Inc.
Lainie Hinnant

4 Runswick Drive
Richmond, VA 23233

Lyme Information Center of
  Virginia
Joan McCullum
P.O. Box 3096
Oakton, VA 22124

National Capital LDA
Monte Skall
7714 Crossover Drive
McLean, VA 22101
703-821-8833
E-mail: NatCapLyme@aol.
  com

WASHINGTON, D.C.
Washington Metro Area LDA
Kenneth Klein
641 Indiana Avenue NW
Washington, DC 20004

WISCONSIN
Fond du Lac Area Support
Kathryn Montgomery
833 Stirling
Fond du Lac, WI 54935
920-921-5588

Lyme Resource Group of South
  Central Wisconsin
Jeannette Wheat
4306 Fawn Court
Cross Plains, WI 53528

608-798-4421
E-mail: NILR@aol.com

Seymour Wisconsin Area SG
Monica Johnson
824 Woodside Drive
Seymour, WI 54165
920-833-2114
E-mail: monicaj@expecpc

International Support Groups

CANADA
Lyme Borreliosis Support Group
  of Manitoba
Elizabeth Wood
350 Rougeau Avenue
Winnipeg, Manitoba R2C 4A2,
  Canada

Lyme Disease Association of
  Ontario
John Scott
365 St. David Street South
Fergus, Ontario N1M 2L7,
  Canada

Lyme Disease Society of
  Saskatchewan
Melanie Chernipeski
P.O. Box 7
Tugaske, Saskatchewan
  SOH 4BO, Canada

Lyme Disease Support Group of
  New Brunswick
Linda Dochstader
106 Carriage Hill Drive
Fredericton, New Brunswick
  E3E 1A4, Canada

Nova Scotia Lyme Borreliosis
  Support Group
Edna MacNeil
P.O. Box 1540
4 Maple Street
Pictou, Nova Scotia BOK 1HO,
  Canada

Vancouver BC Lyme B
  Society
Diane Kindree
P.O. Box 91535
W. Vancouver, British Columbia
  V7V 3P2, Canada

GERMANY
German Support Group
  Information
Peter Rohleder
+49-2241-142208
E-mail: peter.rohleder@
  gmd.de

NETHERLANDS
Dutch Lyme Disease Patient
  Organization
Brianstraat 50 6372 Be
Landgraaf, Netherlands

European Lyme Foundation
Schiekade 404
3032 AX
Rotterdam, Netherlands

UNITED KINGDOM
British Lyme Disease Foundation
Mark Greenfield
P.O. Box 110
Tunbridge Wells
Kent, England TN1 1WY

The Lyme Society
Mrs. G. S. Reese
4 Thorpe, Leys

Lockington, Driffield
East York, England
  Y025 9SP

SPAIN
Spanish Lyme Support
  Group
Miguel Angel Ramirez
E-mail: yolandadiaz
  @jazzfee.com
Mr. Ramirez is fluent in English
  as well as Spanish.
Spanish support group e-mail:
  lyme_y_otras_zoonsis_cronicas
  _espanol@yahoogroups.com

Appendix C:
Helpful Links and Websites

America On Lyme
http://members.aol.com/americaonlyme/aolyme

American Lyme Disease Foundation
Mill Pond offices
293 Route 100
Somers, NY 10589
914-277-6970
E-mail: Inquire@aldf.com
www.aldf.com

Bowen Research and Training Institute
38541 U.S. Highway 19 North
Palm Harbor, FL 34684
Dr. Jo Anne Whitaker, President and Director
727-937-9877
http://www.bowen.org

FAMILIES USA—Health Assistance Partnership
Assistance with insurance issues
1334 G Street NW
Washington, DC 20005
202-737-6340
http://www.healthassistancepartnership.org

International Lyme and Associated Diseases Society (ILADS)
Professional medical and research organization
P.O. Box 341461
Bethesda, MD 20827
http://www.ilads.org

Lyme Alliance, Inc.
Spotlight on Lyme newsletter, medical information, and more
P.O. Box 454
Concord, MI 49237
Sharon Smith, President
E-mail: barbfitz@chartermi.net

Lyme Disease Association (LDA)
Excellent up-to-date information, news, resources, referrals, links,
    support
5019 Megill Road
Farmingdale, NJ 07727
Pat Smith, President
732-938-4834
E-mail: lymeliter@aol.com
http://www.lymediseaseassociation.org

Lyme Disease Association of Ohio
Carol Long, President
614-475-8960
E-mail: lymecare@aol.com

Lyme Disease Coalition of Minnesota
Lynn Olivier, President
902 Grandview Avenue
Duluth, MN 55812
218-728-3914
E-mail: lymenet_mn@yahoo.com
http://olivierlynn.freeyellow.com/LD-Coalition_MN

Lyme Disease Foundation
1 Financial Plaza
Hartford, CT 06103
E-mail: lymefnd@aol.com
http://www.Lyme.org

Lyme Disease Information Resource
Information, Internet links, and other patient resources
http://www.healingwell.com/pages/LymeDisease

Lyme Disease Network
Information about diagnosis and treatment of Lyme,
    affiliate of LDA
43 Winton Road
East Brunswick, NJ 08816
E-mail: bill@LymeNet.org
http://lymenet.org

Lyme Disease Resource Center (LDRC)
An affiliate of the Lyme Disease Association, Inc., LDRC is a non-profit organization founded in 1990 by a group of individuals who had personal experience with Lyme disease and wanted to help people who were going undiagnosed because doctors were not well informed about this newly emerging infection.
http://www.Lymedisease.org/pacificLyme

Lyme Research and Practice (formerly the Lyme Project)
Dr. Daniel J. Cameron
Mt. Kisco, NY 10549
914-666-4665
E-mail: cameron@lymeproject.com
http://lymeproject.com

Massachusetts Lyme Disease Coalition of Cape Cod Lyme Disease Awareness Association
John Coughlan, President
P.O. Box 1916
Mashpee, MA 02649
508-563-7033

Medscape AE
Features full-text, peer-reviewed articles, MEDLINE, and interactive
   quizzes; updated daily
http://www.medscape.com

Michigan Lyme Disease Association
Linda Lobes, President
888-784-5963 (toll-free)
E-mail: Lpurdy1040@aol.com
http://www.homestead.com/MichiganLymeDiseaseAssoc/
   mldahome.html

National Health Institute of Allergy and Infectious Diseases (NIAID)
http://www.niaid.nih.gov/

NeedyMeds.com
P.O. Box 63716
Philadelphia, PA 19147
Dr. Richard Sagall, Libby Overly, founders
215-625-9609 (Do not call with individual problems; check website)
http://www.needymeds.com

NIH/NLM: MEDLINEplus: Lyme Disease
http://medlineplus.nlm.nih.gov/medlineplus/lymedisease.html

Parents of Children with Lyme Disease
Excellent, informative site
Cyntha Landon, chair
http://www.pocwl.org

Time For Lyme, Inc.
Affiliate of LDA
P.O. Box 31269
Greenwich, CT 06831
Diane Blanchard and Debbie Siciliano, co-chairs
203-969-1333
http://www.TimeForLyme.org

Undersea and Hyperbaric Medical Society
UHMS members are scientists and physicians in the field of hyper-
baric medicine.
10531 Metropolitan Avenue
Kensington, MD 20895
Don Chandler, executive director, ext. 101
301-942-2980
E-mail: uhms@uhms.org

University of Rhode Island Tick Research Lab
Information on Lyme and other tick-borne diseases; photos of ticks
http://www.northeastipm/states/ri/#tick

Your Medical Source
Produced by Health Information Publications
http://www.YourMedicalSource.com

International Websites

British Lyme Disease Foundation
Mark Greenfield
P.O. Box 331
East Grinstead, West Sussex
England RH191YT
E-mail: spud@wadhurst.demon.co.uk
http://www.wadhurst.demon.co.uk

Eurolyme—UK and Europe
Gill Reese
E-mail: gilly848@ntlworld.com
http://groups.yahoo.com/group/EuroLyme/

European Union Concerted Action on Lyme Borreliosis (EUCALB)
http://www.dis.strath.ac.uk/vie/LymeEU/index.htm

Lyme Disease Association of Ontario
John D. Scott, President
365 St. David Street South
Fergus, Ontario N1M 2L7, Canada
519-843-3646
www.canlyme.com

Lyme Disease Society of Saskatchewan
Melanie Chernipeski
P.O. Box 7
Tugaske, Saskatchewan SOH 4BO, Canada
306-759-2880
E-mail: lymedisease@asaktel.net

World International Lyme Disease Emergency Rescue (WILDER)
  Network
P.O. Box 116
Forestville, CA 95436
http://www.wildernetwork.org/index.html

Articles, Conference Summaries, and Biographies Online

Fallon et al., "Late-Stage Neuropsychiactric Lyme Borelliosis"
http://www.columbia-/Lyme.org

Fallon et al., "The Neuropsychiactric Manifestation of Lyme Borelliosis"
http://www.columbia-/Lyme.org

Journal of Spirochetal and Tick-borne Diseases
http://www.slackinc.com/general/jstd/jstdhome.htm

Liegner, K., "Lyme Disease: The Sensible Pursuit of Answers"
http://www.lymenet.org

Active Studies and Clinical Trials

Chronic Lyme Disease Study

An NIH-funded study under the auspices of Columbia University
College of Physicians and Surgeons
Director: Dr. Brian A. Fallon
Coordinator: Dr. Kathy Corbera
212-543-6510
E-mail: CULyme@aol.com
http://www.columbia-lyme.org
Purpose of the study is to answer critical scientific questions about the
treatment and cause of persistent Lyme symptoms. Eligibility: age
18–65 with a well-documented history of Lyme that meets CDC criteria and a currently positive IgG Western blot or Lyme PCR; treatment
of more than 4 months, with at least 3 weeks of IV antibiotics. Must
be willing to travel to Columbia University in New York City four
times during a one-year period.

Lyme Disease Study

National Institute of Allergy and Infectious Diseases (NIAID)
Patient Recruitment and Public Liaison Office
Bethesda, Maryland
800-411-1222 (toll-free)
E-mail: prpl@mail.cc.nih.gov
http://www.niaid.nih.gov
Purpose of the study is to establish a population of patients with
Lyme disease for evaluation, treatment, and follow-up to learn more
about the infection. Eligibility: patients with active Lyme disease who
have a medical history and physical examination and diagnostic

evaluations appropriate to their individual condition. No experimental procedures will be offered under this protocol. Patients will be followed as needed for evaluation and treatment of their condition. In general, they will be asked to return at the end of therapy; then 3, 6, and 12 months later; and then every 6 to 12 months.

The Retreatment Study
Director: Dr. Daniel Cameron
914-666-4665
E-mail: Comments@LymeProject.com
http://www.lymeproject.com
Clinical trial designed to see how the drug amoxicillin compares to placebo in resolving recurrent Lyme disease in patients who were initially successfully treated. Eligibility: age 18 or older with initial successful treatment of Lyme. Volunteers are not eligible to participate if they are allergic to amoxicillin or have failed amoxicillin therapy in the past. Must be willing to travel to Mt. Kisco, New York, for multiple assessments.

Appendix D:
Active Newsletters

Some of these newsletters are free; others have a subscription fee. Contact the publication for information.

Bulls'eye
Greater Cleveland Lyme Disease Support Group
Ann Hirschberg, Editor
7644 Main Street
Cleveland, OH 44138
216-235-4463
E-mail: Gcldsg@aol.com

Lyme Alert
Lyme Disease Association of Ontario
365 St. David Street South
Fergus, Ontario N1M 2L7, Canada
519-843-3646

Lyme Community News
Lyme Disease Coalition
401 Baker Lane
Coatesville, PA 19320-2205
610-384-9622
E-mail: Lyme911@aol.com

Lyme Disease Education Project
(Patient/physician perspectives from the U.S. and Canada)
Lora Mermin, Editor
321 Palomino Lane, #2 South
Madison, WI 53705
608-231-2199

Lyme Disease Update
Angela M. Salm, Editor
P.O. Box 15711-0711
Evansville, IN 47716
812-471-1990

Lyme Letter
Westchester Lyme Support Group
Mark Kramer
P.O. Box 82
Irvington, NY 10533
914-591-7023

Lymelight
Chris Malinowski, Editor
Lyme Disease Foundation
One Financial Plaza
Hartford, CT 06103
860-525-2000 or 800-886-LYME
E-mail: lymefnd@aol.com
http://www.Lyme.org

Lyme Matters
An online newsletter e-mailed weekly and monthly, free.
Send your e-mail address to PSPatches@aol.com asking to subscribe.
http://www.angelfire.com/ny/lymedisease/mattersmain.html

LymeSig
Dave Bartholomew, Editor/Publisher
323 Chapel Avenue
Allentown, PA 18103-3457
610-797-3229
E-mail: JRQR18A@prodigy.com
http://ourworld.compuserve.com/homcpages/frankd/Lymesig.htm

The Lyme Times
Lyme Disease Resource Center
Phyllis Mervine, Editor
P.O. Box 707
Weaverville, CA 96093
E-mail: Info@lymedisease.org

Lyme Treatment News
National Lyme Community Research Institute
Richard Lynch, Editor
17 Monroe Avenue
Staten Island, NY 10301
718-273-3740

Spotlight on Lyme
Lyme Alliance, Inc.
Sharon Smith and Maria Current, Editors
P.O. Box 454
Concord, MI 49237
http://www.lymealliance.org/newsletter

the ticked-off tract
Laura Ames, Editor/Publisher
325 Fresno Street
Coalinga, CA 93210
209-935-0914

Bibliography

Alexander, Ames. "Profit Motive Alleged in Lyme Disease Care." *Asbury Park Press,* 29 March 1992.

"A Model Plan." *The Fresno Bee,* 5 September 1990.

Appel, Max J. G. "Lyme Disease in Dogs and Cats." In *The Compendium,* Ithaca, N.Y.: Cornell University, May 1990.

Asbrink, Eva, and Anders Hovmark. "Early and Late Cutaneous Manifestations in Ixodes-borne Borreliosis (Erythema Migrans Borreliosis, Lyme Borreliosis)." *Annals of the New York Academy of Sciences,* 1989.

Bakken, Lori L., et al. "Performance of 45 Laboratories Participating in a Proficiency Testing Program for Lyme Disease Serology." *Journal of the American Medical Association,* 19 August 1992, pp. 891–95.

Barrett, Katherine, and Richard Green. "How to Get the Most from Your Health Insurance." *Ladies' Home Journal,* June 1992, p. 52.

Battelle, Phyllis. "My Doctor Said I Had AIDS—I Didn't." *Redbook,* March 1992.

Belkin, Lisa. "In Lessons on Empathy, Doctors Become Patients." *New York Times,* 4 June 1992.

Blackburn, Norris. "Lyme Disease: A Serious Threat." *Blue Ridge Outdoors,* October 1992, pp. 16–17.

Bleiweiss, John. "When to Suspect Lyme Disease." *The Lyme Threat.* American Lyme Disease Alliance, Fall 1992.

Bowen, G. Stephen, Terry L. Schulze, and William Parkin. "Lyme Disease in New Jersey, 1978–1982." *Yale Journal of Biology & Medicine,* 1984, pp. 661–68.

Bozsik, Bela P., et al. "Combined Antiobitic Treatment of Lyme Borreliosis." Abstract 67, V *International Conference on Lyme Borreliosis.* Arlington, Va.: May 1992.

Brataas, Anne. "Living with Lyme Disease." *St. Paul Express,* 16 May 1992.

Brenner, Carl. "Lyme Disease: Asking the Right Questions." *Science* 257 (25 September 1992).

Brody, Jane. "Dealing with Lyme Disease Can Be a Tough Call." *New York Times,* 26 August 1992.

———. "For Time Outdoors, Ways to Avoid Lyme Disease." *New York Times,* 26 June 1991.

Brorson, O., S. H. Brorson. "In Vitro Conversion of *Borrelia burgdorferi* to Cystic Forms in Spinal Fluid, and Transformation to Mobile Spirochetes by Incubation in BSK-H Medium." *Infection* 2 (February 1998).

Bukro, Casey. "Lyme Borreliosis: Ten Years after Discovery of the Etiologic Agent, *Borrelia burgdorferi.*" *Infection,* Special reprint, vol. 19 (1991):3–7.

———. "Lyme Disease Presents Threat to Woodlands Hikers, Campers." *Chicago Tribune,* 16 June 1991.

Burgdorfer, Willy. "Discovery of the Lyme Disease Spirochete: A Historical Review." *International Journal of Microbiology and Hygiene,* Series A, Medical Microbiology, Infectious Diseases, Virology, Parasitology, 1986, pp. 7–9.

———. "Lyme Borreliosis: Ten Years after Discovery of the Etiologic Agent, *Borrelia burgdorferi.*" *Infection,* Special reprint, vol. 19 (1991):3–7.

Burrascano, Joseph, Jr. "Advanced Topics in Lyme Disease," November 2002, 14th ed.

Burrascano, Joseph J., Jr. "Diagnostic Hints and Treatment Guidelines for Lyme Disease." October 1991. Pamphlet.

———. Letter. *Internal Medicine World Report,* 10 December 1991.

———. "Late Stage Lyme Disease: Treatment Options and Guidelines." *Internal Medicine* 10 (December 1989).

———. "Lyme Disease Rehabilitation." Treatment paper guidelines, presented at Lyme Disease Consensus Meeting, November 1992.

————. "Managing Lyme Disease: Diagnostic Hints and Treatment Guidelines for Lyme Borreliosis." Tenth edition, February 1995. Pamphlet.

————. "Transmission of *Borrelia burgdorferi* by Blood Transfusion." Abstract 256A, *V International Conference on Lyme Borreliosis.* Arlington, Va.: May 1992.

Burstein, Edward. "Coping, or Not Coping, with Stress." *UC the Independent Press,* 8 January 1992, p. 11.

Cameron, Daniel J., and Victoria P. Malara. "Successful Retreatment of Lyme." Abstract 70C, *V International Conference on Lyme Borreliosis.* Arlington, Va.: May 1992.

Cartter, Matthew L., et al. "Epidemiology of Lyme Disease in Connecticut." *Connecticut Medicine,* June 1989, pp. 320–23.

Cassem, Edwin H. "When Symptoms Seem Groundless." *Emergency Medicine,* 15 June 1992, pp. 191–99.

Cavert, Kathy. "Lyme Disease—United States." *Morbidity and Mortality Weekly Report,* 2 October 1992, pp. 726–27.

CDC. "Epidemiologic Notes and Reports on Babesiosis—Connecticut." *MMWR Weekly,* 38 (28 September 1989):649–50.

————. "Lyme Disease-United States, 2000," *MMWR Weekly,* 51 (18 January 2002):29–30.

————. "Southern Tick-Associated Rash Illness." Division of Vector-Borne Diseases, National Center for Infectious Diseases, 15 October 2001.

Centers for Disease Control, Morbidity and Mortality Weekly Report. "Effectiveness in Disease and Injury Prevention: Lyme Disease Knowledge, Attitudes, and Behaviors—Connecticut, 1992." *Archives of Dermatology* 128 (September 1992):1171.

————. "Lyme Disease Questionnaire." Midwest Lyme Disease Association, November 1990.

————. "Lyme Disease Surveillance Case Definition." Program for prevention and control of Lyme disease, 1992.

————. "Surviving Lyme Disease." *LymeAid,* June/July 1992.

Clark, Jane R., et al. "Facial Paralysis in Lyme Disease." *Laryngoscope,* November 1985.

Classen, Norma. "Lyme Disease Easiest to Cure When Diagnosed,

Treated in Early Stages." *University Chronicle.* St. Cloud State University, 24 March 1992.

Coyle, P. K. "Neurologic Lyme Disease." *Seminars in Neurology* 12 (September 1992):2–10.

Crist, Charles L. "Pulse Therapy with Antibiotic Needs More Research." *Lyme Disease Update,* November 1991.

Dattwyler, Raymond J. "Lyme Borreliosis: An Overview of the Clinical Manifestations." *Laboratory Medicine* 21 (May 1990):290–92.

Devery, Glenn. "Lyme Disease: A Tick(ing) Bomb." *Outdoor Life,* February 1988, p. 42.

Dinerman, Hal, and Allen Steere. "Lyme Disease Associated with Fibromyalgia." *Annals of Internal Medicine,* August 1992.

Doepel, Laurie K. "NIAID Scientists Develop Direct Method to Detect Presence of the Lyme Disease Spirochete." *Update,* April 1991.

Doepel, Laurie K., and Barbara Weldon. "Researchers Battle Lyme Disease." *Healthline,* June 1991.

Drulle, John. "Lyme Disease: Late Season Update." *Drug Therapy* 25 (August 1989):36–42.

———. "Pregnancy and Lyme Disease." *LymeAid,* August/September 1990.

Drummon, Roger. "Ticks and What You Can Do about Them." Berkeley, Calif.: Wilderness Press, 1990.

Durkin, Barbara J. "New Way Found to Test for Lyme." *The Reporter Dispatch* (Westchester County, N.Y.), 9 September 1992, p. 9.

———. "Spinal Tap Helps Doctor Spot Infection." *The Reporter Dispatch* (Westchester County, N.Y.), 18 May 1992.

Edelman, Robert. "Perspective on the Development of Vaccines against Lyme Disease." *Vaccine* 9 (August 1991):531–32.

Ellis, B. J. "The Threat of Lyme Disease." *Columbia Metropolitan* 89 (July/August 1992):339–42.

Etling, Kathy. "Lyme Disease: What Makes It Tick." *Outdoor Life,* May 1990, p. 43.

European Union Concerted Action on Lyme Borreliosis (EUCALB). "Risk: Epidemiology of European Lyme Borreliosis," 30 May 2003.

Fallon, Brian A., and Jennifer Nields. "Lyme Disease: A Neuropsychiatric Illness." *American Journal of Psychiatry* 151 (November 1994):1571–83.

Fallon, Brian A., et al. "The Neuropsychiatric Manifestations of Lyme Borreliosis." *Psychiatric Quarterly* 63 (Spring 1992):95–117.

———. "The Underdiagnosis of Neuropsychiatric Lyme Disease in Children and Adults." *Psychiatric Clinics of North America* 21 (September 1998).

Feaga, Wendy P. *Handbook on Lyme Borreliosis.* 4th ed. Ellicott City, Md., June 1991.

Fernandez, Ana, and Leonard Sigal. "Trends in the Therapy of Lyme Disease." *Today's Therapeutic Trends.* University of Medicine and Dentistry of NJ, Robert Wood Johnson Medical School, 1992.

Fife, W. P., and D. M. Freeman. "The Use of Hyperbaric Oxygen Therapy for the Treatment of Lyme Disease." Texas A&M University.

Finn, Albert F., Jr., and Raymond J. Dattwyler. "The Immunology of Lyme Borreliosis." *Laboratory Medicine* 21 (May 1990):305.

Flach, Allan J., and Paul E. Lavoie. "Episcleritis, Conjunctivitis, and Keratitis as Ocular Manifestations of Lyme Disease." *Ophthalmology* 97 (August 1990):973–75.

Freedman, Mitchell. "Ticks Get No Shelter on Island." *Newsday,* 7 July 1991.

Friedman, Emily. "Insurers under Fire." *HMQ,* Third Quarter 1991, p. 23.

Garcia-Monco, Juan C., et al. "*Borrelia burgdorferi* in the Central Nervous System: Experimental and Clinical Evidence for Early Invasion." *Journal of Infectious Disease,* June 1990, pp. 1187–93.

Georgilis, Kostis, M. Peacocke, and M. S. Klempner. "Fibroblasts Protect the Lyme Disease Spirochete, *Borrelia burgdorferi,* from Ceftriaxone in Vitro." *Journal of Infectious Disease,* August 1992, pp. 440–44.

Gerber, Michael A., et al. "Risk of Acquiring Lyme Disease or Babesiosis from a Blood Transfusion in Connecticut," Abstract 361, *V International Conference on Lyme Borreliosis.* Arlington, Va.: May 1992.

Gerber, Paul C. "How to Hold Third-Party Payers Accountable for

Second-Guessing You." *Physician's Management,* December 1990, p. 23.

Gerlin, Andrea. "Lyme Disease Spurs Disputes over Treatment." *The Wall Street Journal,* 28 July 1992.

Graham, Tom. "Lyme and Punishment; A Weekly Check on Health Care Costs and Coverage." *Washington Post,* 12 August 2003.

Hall, R. D., et al. "Research on Ticks and Tick-borne Pathogens in Missouri—An Interim Research Report." *Missouri Medicine* 89 (June 1991):339–42.

Hassler, Dieter, et al. Letter. "Pulsed High-Dose Cefotaxime Therapy in Refractory Lyme Borreliosis." *The Lancet* 338 (20 July 1991):193.

Hearn, Wayne. "Expert Witness Sued for Giving His Opinion during Peer Review." *American Medical News,* 11 May 1992, p. 3.

Heltzel, Jo Ann. *Learning about Lyme Disease.* Woodbury, Minn.: privately published, 1991.

Jaffe, Herb. "Blues File Suit against Health Care Firms, MD and Others in $4 Million Bilk." *The Star Ledger* (Newark, N.J.), 14 September 1992.

Johns, Stephanie. "Doctors' Favorite Doctors." *New Jersey Monthly,* April 1992, pp. 42–46.

Kantor, Fred S. "Disarming Lyme Disease." *Scientific American,* September 1994, pp. 34–37.

Katzel, James H. "Is There a Consensus in Treatment of Lyme Borreliosis?" Paper presented at the Lyme Borreliosis Foundation International Symposium in California, April 1991.

———. "What Is the Best Treatment for Lyme Borreliosis (Lyme Disease)?" *the ticked-off tract,* October 1992.

———. "What Type of Doctor Treats Lyme Disease?" *the ticked-off tract,* November 1992.

Katzel, James H., and Ross I. Ritter. "Lyme Disease without Erythema Migrans, Five Case Studies." Abstract 55C, *V International Conference on Lyme Borreliosis.* Arlington, Va.: May 1992.

Keller, Tracey L., J. J. Halperin, and M. Whitman. "PCR Detection of *Borrelia burgdorferi* DNA in Cerebrospinal Fluid of Lyme Neuroborreliosis Patients." *Neurology,* January 1992, pp. 32–34.

Khare, Madan L. "Lyme Disease Forum: Peril for Household Pets." *The Messenger-Press* (New Jersey), 25 July 1991.

Kong, Delores. "Swift Treatment Urged to Avert Lyme Disease." *The Boston Globe*, 20 August 1992.

Lavoie, Paul E. "Failure of Published Antibiotic Regimens in L. Borreliosis: Observations on Prolonged Oral Therapy." Paper presented at the Lyme Borreliosis International Conference, Sweden, 1990.

———. "Lyme Disease." *Conn's Current Therapy*, 1991.

———. "Lyme Disease: Pregnancy." *Rakel's Current Therapy*, 1991.

Leary, Warren E. "Exhibition Examines Scientists' Complicity in Nazi-Era Atrocities." *New York Times*, 10 November 1992, p. C3.

Liegner, Kenneth. "Minocycline in Lyme Disease." *Journal of the American Academy of Dermatology* 28 (January 1993):131.

———. "Remarks Before the NYS Assembly Committee on Health." Albany, New York, 27 November 2001.

Liegner, Kenneth B., et al. "Culture-Confirmed Treatment Failure of Cefotaxim and Minocycline in a Case of Lyme Meningoencephalomyelitis in the United States." Abstract 63, *V International Conference on Lyme Borreliosis*. Arlington, Va.: May 1992.

———. "Recurrent Erythema Migrans Despite Extended Antibiotic Treatment with Minocycline in a Patient with Persisting BB Infection." *M. Dermatology*, August 1992.

Lissman, Barry A., et al. "Spirochete-Associated Arthritis (Lyme Disease) in a Dog." *Journal of the American Veterinary Association* 185 (15 July 1984):219–20.

Loftus, John. *The Belarus Secret: The Nazi Connection in America.* Alfred A. Knopf, New York, 1982.

Logigian, Eric, Richard F. Kaplan, and Allen Steere. "Chronic Neurologic Manifestations of Lyme Disease." *New England Journal of Medicine*, 22 November 1990, pp. 1438–44.

Loutit, Jeffery S. "Bartonella Infections: Diverse and Elusive." *Hospital Practice, Stanford University*, 1998.

Luft, Benjamin J., et al. "Invasion of the Central Nervous System by *Borrelia burgdorferi* in Acute Disseminated Infection." *Journal of the American Medical Association*, 11 March 1992, pp. 1364–67.

"Lyme Disease: Not Just Deer Ticks." *American Health*, June 1989.

"Lyme Disease Clinic to Open." *Shoshone* (Idaho) *News Press,* 19 September 1990.

Lyme Disease Coalition of New Jersey, Inc. "Lyme Disease Patient Position Paper," 1992.

MacDonald, Alan B. "Gestational Lyme Borreliosis Implications for the Fetus." *Rheumatic Disease Clinics of North America,* 15 November 1989.

MacDonald, Alan B., J. L. Benach, and W. Burgdorfer. "Stillbirth Following Maternal Lyme Disease." NY *State Journal of Medicine,* 1987.

Maes, Edith, Pascal Lecomte, and Nancy Ray. "A Cost-of-Illness Study of Lyme Disease in the United States." *Clinical Therapeutics* 20 (1998).

Magid, David, et al. "Prevention of Lyme Disease after Tick Bites: A Cost-Effective Analysis." *New England Journal of Medicine,* 20 August 1992.

Magnarelli, Louis A. "Derologic Diagnosis of Lyme Disease." *Annals, New York Academy of Sciences,* 1 May 1987.

Magnarelli, Louis A., et al. "Antibodies to *Borrelia burgdorferi* in Rodents in the Eastern and Southern United States." *Journal of Clinical Microbiology,* June 1992, pp. 1449–52.

Magnarelli, Louis, and John F. Anderson. "Ticks and Biting Insects Infected with the Etiologic Agent of Lyme Disease, *Borrelia burgdorferi.*" *Journal of Clinical Microbiology,* August 1988, pp. 1482–86.

Marconi, Richard T., W. Hauglum, and Claude F. Garon. "Species-specific Identification of and Distinction between *Borrelia burgdorferi* Genome Groups by Using 16S RNA-Directed Oligonucleotide Probes." *Journal of Clinical Microbiology,* March 1992, pp. 628–32.

Marshall, Eliot. "NIH Gears Up to Test a Hotly Disputed Theory." *Science* 270 (13 October 1995): 228–29.

Marshall, Vincent. "Multiple Sclerosis Is a Chronic Central Nervous System Infection by a Spirochetal Agent." *Medical Hypotheses.* Animal Vaccine Laboratory, 1987.

Massarotti, Elena M., et al. "Treatment of Early Lyme Disease." *American Journal of Medicine,* April 1992, pp. 396–403.

Masters, Edwin J. "Erythema Migrans of Lyme Disease." *The Solution,* Special ed., 1992.

Masters, Edwin J., Pamela Lynxwiler, and Julie Rawlings. "Spirochetemia Two Weeks Post Cessation of Six Months Continuous P.O. Amoxicillin Therapy." Abstract 65, *V International Conference on Lyme Borreliosis.* Arlington, Va.: May 1992.

McCarthy, Laura Flynn. "Far from the Medical Mainstream." *Cosmopolitan,* June 1992, p. 263.

Mermin, Lora, ed. *Lyme Disease 1991: Patient/Physician Perspectives from the U.S. and Canada.* Madison, Wis.: The Lyme Disease Education Project, 1991.

Moran, Stephen J. "Physical, Financial Strain of Lyme Disease Addressed." *The Press of Atlantic City,* 15 November 1992.

Moulton, Chris. "Lyme Disease: New Facts Only Add to Diagnostic Frustrations." *Advance for Med Lab Professionals,* 29 July 1991, pp. 18–19.

Mueller, Mark. "Lyme Disease Infects State." *The Trentonian,* 23 December 1991.

National Institute on Aging. "New Prevalence Study Suggests Dramatically Rising Numbers of People with Alzheimer's Disease." *NIH News,* 18 August 2003.

National Institute of Allergy and Infectious Diseases. "Lyme Disease." *Backgrounder,* June 1991.

National Institutes of Health. "New NIH Research Grants on Lyme Disease." Department of Health and Human Services Fact Sheet, 23 July 1990.

NIH State-of-the-Art Conference. "Diagnosis and Treatment of Lyme Disease." *Clinical Courier 9* (August 1991).

Pachner, Andrew R., and Andrea Itano. "*Borrelia burgdorferi* Infection of the Brain." *Neurology,* October 1990, pp. 1535–40.

Paparone, Philip W. "There Is No Standard Approach to Lyme Disease: Your Management Must Be Individualized." *Modern Medicine* 60 (September 1992):335–37.

Payer, Lynn. *Disease Mongers: How Doctors, Drug Companies, and Insurers Are Making You Feel Sick.* New York: John Wiley & Sons, 1992.

Pfister, H. W., et al. "Latent Lyme Neuroborreliosis: Presence of *Borrelia burgdorferi* in the Cerebrospinal Fluid without Concurrent Inflammatory Signs." *Neurology* 39 (1989):1118–20.

Piesman, Joseph, et al. "Duration of Tick Attachment and *Borrelia burgdorferi* Transmission." *Journal of Clinical Microbiology,* March 1987, pp. 557–58.

Pietrucha, Dorothy M. "Many Difficult Problems for Children with Lyme." *Lyme Times, Newsletter of the LD Resource Center* 3 (Summer 1992).

———. "Neurologic Manifestations of Lyme Disease in Children." Paper presented at the National Lyme B. Scientific Symposium, March 1990.

———. "Neurologic Manifestations, Treatment for Youngsters." *The Messenger Press,* 22 August 1991.

"Pinning Down the Lyme Disease Antibody." *Science News* 137 (1990):156.

Plotkin, Stanley A., and Georges Peter. "Treatment of Lyme Borreliosis." *Pediatrics* 88 (July 1991):176–79.

Post, John E. "Lyme Disease in Large Animals." *Lyme Disease Update,* April 1991.

Preac-Mursic, V., et al. "Survival of *Borrelia burgdorferi* in Antibiotically Treated Patients with Lyme Borreliosis." *Infection* 5 (1989): 355–59.

Rhode Island Department of Health. "Report on the Governor's Commission on Lyme and Other Tick-Borne Illnesses." Providence, Rhode Island, September 2003.

Roberts, E. Donald, et al. "Chronic Lyme Disease in the Rhesus Monkey." *Laboratory Investigation.* US and Canadian Academy of Pathology 72 (1995):146–56.

Schoen, Robert T. "Treatment of Lyme Disease." *Connecticut Medicine* 53 (June 1989):335–37.

Schutzer, Steven E., et al. "Sequestration of Antibody to *Borrelia*

burgdorferi in Immune Complexes in Seronegative Lyme Disease."
The Lancet 335 (10 February 1990):312–15.

Seligmann, Jean, et al. "Lyme Disease: Tiny Tick, Big Worry."
Newsweek, 22 May 1989.

Sigal, Leonard H. "Lyme Disease: Don't Let Its Disguises Fool You."
Internal Medicine 13 (June 1992):24–33.

Steere, Allen C. "Distinguishing Lyme Disease from Its Look-Alikes."
Emergency Medicine, 15 August 1992, pp. 28–44.

Sturmfels, Peg. "Lyme Disease Forum: Parents Must Become Teachers
and Advocates." *The Messenger-Press* (New Jersey), 22 August
1991.

Sullivan, Patricia. "Health Insurers Limit Drugs for Lyme Disease."
The Star Ledger (Newark, N.J.), 22 March 1992.

3M Company. "Employees Are Urged to Be Aware of Lyme Disease."
The Stemwinder, 10 April 1991.

Tager, Felice, et al. "A Controlled Study of Cognitive Deficits in Children with Chronic Lyme Disease." *Journal of Neuropsychiatry and
Clinical Neurosciences* 13 (2001):500–507.

Vanderhoof, Irwin T., and Karen M. B. Vanderhoof-Forschner. "Lyme
Disease: The Cost to Society." Paper prepared as a funded project
for the Lyme Disease Foundation and the Society of Actuaries, July
1992.

———. "Lyme Disease: The Cost to Society." *Contingencies,* Janu-
ary/February 1993, pp. 42–48.

Varde, Shobha, John Beckley, and Ira Schwartz. "Prevalence of Tick-
Borne Pathogens in *Ixodes scapularis* in a Rural New Jersey
County." *Emerging Infectious Diseases* 4 (January–March 1998).

Watson, Linda. "Bringing Up Baby." *Homecare,* September 1992,
p. 41.

Weldon, Barbara. "Dr. Steere Reports on Long-term Effects of Lyme on
Children." *Lyme Times, Newsletter of the LD Resource Center,*
Summer/Fall 1991, p. 15.

———. "Lyme Ticks Hitch Ride on Birds." *Healthline,* June 1991.

Wheat, Jeannette W. "What You Haven't Heard about Lyme Disease."
Wisconsin Pharmacist, July 1991, pp. 16–18.

Whitlow, Joan. "Home Therapy Comes with Price Markups." *Newark Star Ledger,* 29 March 1992.

Wormser, Gary P. "Treatment of *Borrelia burgdorferi* Infection." *Laboratory Medicine* 21 (May 1990):316–21.

Wormser, Gary P., et al. "Use of a Novel Technique of Cutaneous Lavage for Diagnosis of Lyme Disease Associated with Erythema Migrans." *Journal of the American Medical Association,* 9 September 1992, pp. 1311–13.

Acknowledgments

An update of a book as technically and emotionally complex as *Coping With Lyme Disease* could never have been completed without the assistance of many, many special people.

Dr. Kenneth Liegner, my distinguished medical advisor, could be described as a true Renaissance man. Not only has he treated his patients with constantly mined, up-to-the-minute knowledge and grace, but he has been a tireless researcher, a valiant fighter for patients' rights in the trenches and in Washington, and, on top of all this, he plays a mean horn. I am honored that he has taken time from his overloaded schedule to share his expertise and kindness with all the readers of this book.

It has been my great privilege to have been the beneficiary of the generosity of time, knowledge, and experience of physicians like Dr. Brian Fallon, Dr. Charles Ray Jones, Dr. Richard Horowitz, Dr. Dorothy Pietrucha, and Dr. Joseph Burrascano. All of these dedicated professionals epitomize the term *healer,* and their commitment to curing their patients supersedes any personal comfort, peer criticism, or monetary gain. They are truly the ideal.

I am immensely grateful to Pat Smith of the Lyme Disease Association, whose devoted efforts to further knowledge about Lyme and relieve suffering drives her to spend ungodly hours in the service of others—for all of our benefit. Special thanks also go to Debbie Siciliano and Diane Blanchard of *Time For Lyme* in Greenwich, Connecticut, and Barbara Brennan in North Carolina. They have proven that motivation can move mountains.

I must sadly acknowledge the passing of several people who fought the good fight for Lyme disease and taught me about advocacy: Betty Gross, New York, who founded the first Lyme support group in the country; Kathy Cavert, Missouri, who founded the Midwest Lyme Disease Association; and Dr. John Bleiwiess, New Jersey, who years ago pioneered administering combination antibiotics. Their work and their selflessness has, and will, have an impact on the lives of thousands. They are sorely missed. I have chosen to keep their experience and wisdom included in the book.

I thank my daughter Tiffany, who not only experienced life from the inside of a Lyme family, but who, as a communications professional, assisted me in meeting a tight deadline. And thanks to my husband, Alan, who has wrapped his heart, talent, and support around the cause in many ways.

Finally, my hat's off to the many support group leaders, researchers, Lyme-knowledgeable health professionals and education specialists who are touching so many people's lives every day in a positive way. Some are mentioned here; many are not. All are thanked.

Index

About the Authors

DENISE LANG is a popular speaker on family and health issues who has appeared on television shows nationally. An award-winning author and reporter, she currently works as a television producer in New York. She lives in Bridgewater, New Jersey.

KENNETH LIEGNER, M.D., has published articles about Lyme disease in the *Journal of the American Academy of Dermatology, The Journal of Spirochetal and Tick-borne Diseases,* the *New England Journal of Medicine,* and the *Journal of Clinical Microbiology.* He practices medicine in Armonk, New York.